Seizing Control

SEIZING CONTROL

MANAGING EPILEPSY
AND OTHERS'
REACTIONS TO IT
a memoir

LAURA
BERETSKY

*foreword by Steven Schachter, MD
Harvard Medical School*

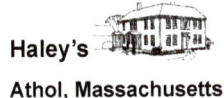

Haley's

Athol, Massachusetts

Copy edited by Ellen Woodbury.

Medusa ornament by Amelia Beretsky-Jewell.

Cover drawing by Susan Gershon.

International Standard Book Number, trade paperback: 978-1-948380-96-6

International Standard Book Number, ePub: 978-1-948380-97-3

International Standard Book Number, Kindle: 978-1-948380-98-0

Haley's

488 South Main Street

Athol, MA 01331

marcia2gagliardi@gmail.com

Library of Congress Cataloging-in-Publication Data

For anybody who has faced the challenges of managing a chronic health condition or a long-term recovery, especially those with refractory epilepsy.

And for my children, Liam and Amelia.

If they don't give you a seat at the table,
bring a folding chair.
—Congresswoman Shirley A. Chisholm
November 30, 1924 – January 1, 2005

Contents

Elevating Awareness about what Epilepsy Is and Isn't
a foreword by Steven C. Schachter, MD

If you have epilepsy, you know that your life is affected by epilepsy much more than you can describe to your doctor during office visits. Indeed, life is lived in the endless stream of moments that we consciously experience day in and day out, and that is way too much to talk about during typically short office visits. It's no wonder, then, that some doctors may not fully appreciate the totality of the lived experience of their patients with epilepsy.

If you have epilepsy, then you also know how epilepsy is stigmatized. It's been that way for centuries. Stigma results from fear and lack of understanding.

For both those reasons, *Seizing Control • managing epilepsy and others' reactions to it* is so remarkable. It presents the author's life in a continuous story and first person account except for the minutes she spent unconscious from seizures. That is how the author has truly lived with epilepsy. She describes her life in such detail that you can almost picture a movie of her life and the endless effects that epilepsy had on her. At the same time, her book removes all misunderstandings about what she experiences with her epilepsy and what she doesn't.

Seizing Control is Laura Beretsky's truth. She bravely shares it with all readers to elevate their awareness about what epilepsy is and isn't and with readers living with epilepsy in the hope that they develop the courage to take as much control of their lives as possible. And she shares it with doctors in the hope that they will work more diligently to understand as much as possible about how epilepsy affects their patients' lives. I would further hope that to accomplish that, doctors would be able to spend enough time with their patients to develop the level of detail depicted by the author. How else can doctors know best how to help people with epilepsy live free of seizures and up to their full potential?

Dr. Schachter, professor of neurology, Harvard Medical School, Boston is chief academic officer for CIMIT, a network of academic and medical institutions partnering with industry and government and a professor of neurology at Harvard Medical School. Past president of the American Epilepsy Society, he has served on the board of directors of the Epilepsy Foundation of America. Dr. Schachter has published more than 250 articles and chapters and edited or written more than 40 books.

Personal Experiences of Epilepsy and Reactions to It
a preface by Laura Beretsky

This is a true story about how I have personally experienced epilepsy and reactions to it.

Epilepsy is a brain disorder that causes recurring, unprovoked seizures. Seizures are sudden surges of abnormal and excessive electrical brain activity that can affect how a person appears or acts.

Seizure symptoms vary widely, depending on the type of seizure. Some seizure signs and symptoms include temporary confusion, staring spells, muscle stiffening, loss of consciousness or awareness, and uncontrollable jerking movements of the limbs. Almost half of the 3.4 million Americans with epilepsy can trace it to a specific cause, including head trauma, brain abnormalities, genetic influence, or prenatal injuries. For the other half, including me, epilepsy is idiopathic, meaning it has no identifiable cause.

I describe incidents based on recollections supplemented by a boatload of my copious notes, email trails, and medical records. Using the pseudonym MEDUSA for my former employer to avoid liability, I factually and accurately describe workplace discrimination. The acronym stands for Make Everything Dandy USA.

I have anchored my professional background in the nonprofit world, typically comprised of mostly well-intentioned staff members dedicated to noble missions. Nevertheless, in my experience, even good-hearted people working at organizations with laudable goals got scared when they witnessed epileptic seizures. Their fears sometimes led to inappropriate responses. I lost out on multiple job opportunities due to my epilepsy. The pseudonym

MEDUSA captures the dichotomy. Upon leaving MEDUSA, I signed an agreement stating I would not share information about their discriminatory workplace practices. I have removed the real MEDUSA from my LinkedIn profile.

Compelled to write this story, I wanted readers to know what a bear it is to manage epilepsy and others' reactions to it. Seizures are scary to observe, and epilepsy has millennia worth of stigma attached, adding to witnesses' fears and negative associations. Whenever I had seizures in others' presence, it worried me far more to imagine subsequent explanations likely required of me than the experience of the seizures themselves. I knew what it took to recover from a complex partial seizure. I wasn't sure what others in my social orbits—friends, family members, colleagues, passersby, dates—might think about me after witnessing me in the throes of one.

I have written a book about the challenges of epilepsy and understand that anybody who manages a perceptible medical condition while trying to fit in and appear "normal" faces their own challenges. The World Health Organization says fifteen percent of the world's population has a disability. I suspect each of us knows and likely loves at least one person who manages a chronic condition.

Passed in 1990, the Americans with Disabilities Act or ADA provides a critical advocacy tool used to help those of us with disabilities fight discriminatory practices and integrate into mainstream life. I am grateful to the disability rights community's tireless advocacy that established the ADA, so others and I could rely upon it. But my journey with epilepsy taught me that the fundamental goal of the ADA cannot be achieved without a major cultural shift that increases society's tolerance, empathy, and courage in the face of people's differences.

I also hope my story empowers patients to collaborate with their medical providers by sharing their symptoms and side effects with them. Playing an active role in one's own healing and healthcare management critically affects a patient's well-being. My story includes descriptions of dozens of doctors' appointments and hospital visits. I used factual dates from medical records. I base exchanges with my providers on my extensive notes and recollections. To protect their confidentiality, I've opted not to include my practitioners' names. My treatment plan included some glitches, but I did not write my story to gain sympathy or vilify my doctors. I've reached out to many of them to thank them for their care, which changed my life.

Regardless of diagnosis, our doctors' textbook knowledge and hands-on experience prove critical to patients' well-being. Knowledge and experience represent only part of the equation for obtaining excellent care. Especially during the COVID-19 era, appointments sometimes occur online. When in-person, appointments often last only for a short time as doctors share their attention with computer screens. Given modern-day arrangements, patients must go to their appointments armed with lists of symptoms and questions to discuss with their practitioners. While our doctors' expertise is essential, patients are our own best experts when it comes to what's going on in our bodies. Ensuring optimal treatment plans depends on each patient's strong self-advocacy.

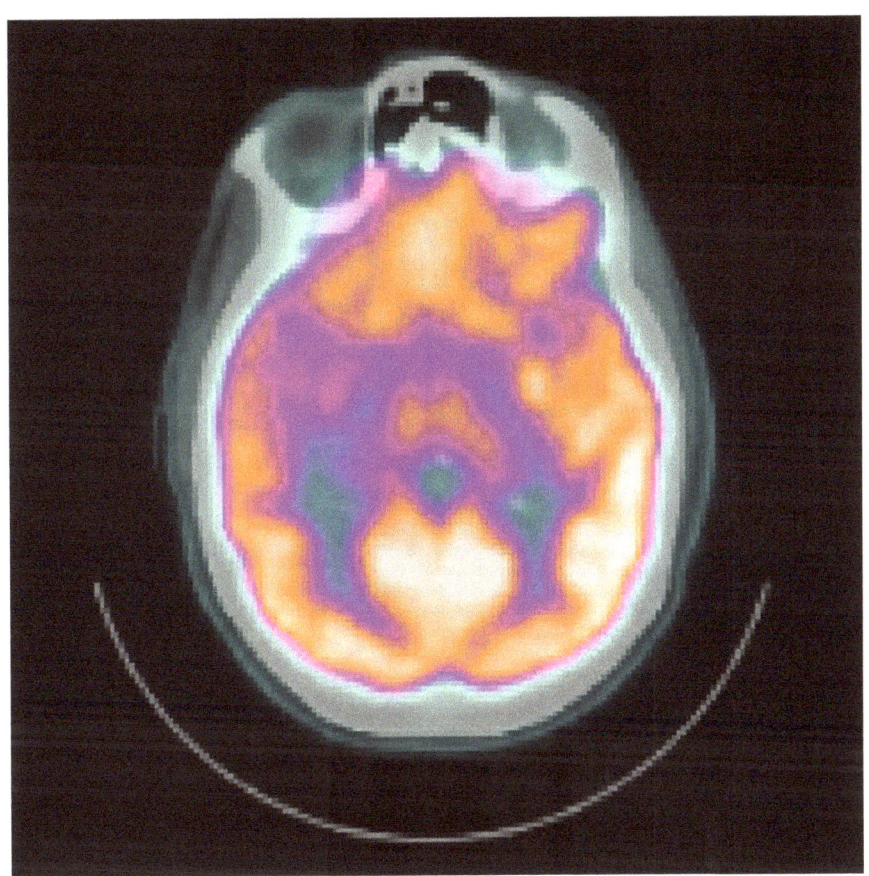

A PET scan shows an image of the author's brain in 2013.

PET SCAN

A PET scan or positron emission tomography shows the brain's use of oxygen or glucose, according to the Epilepsy Foundation.

A very low, safe dose of a radioactive substance is injected into the arm, according to the Epilepsy Foundation, and the scanner records how it travels through the brain. Not all types of PET scans look alike, but often different colors show areas of higher or lower use of oxygen or sugar. The test can help identify the area of the brain where partial seizures arise. It may be done in the period between seizures, called the interictal period.

Professional Consequences

February 2006

Nothing could prepare me for what awaited me when I stepped into Katherine's office. My manager wore a brown pantsuit, the occasional unruly lock of hair diminishing the formal effect. Resting her elbows on a stack of papers as I settled into the chair across from her for our biweekly meeting, Katherine sat at a small round table. She peered at me through her tortoise-shell glasses and cleared her throat.

"Laura, I have to file a disciplinary complaint against you."

She handed me the top pages from her pile. I glanced down, but I couldn't read beyond the bold words "disciplinary action." This didn't make sense. Just the previous month we'd discussed expanding my job responsibilities. I took a deep breath and carefully chose my words.

"I'm surprised—your feedback in my November evaluation was quite positive."

"Yes, but there have been some concerns raised by program managers since then."

Katherine shifted in her seat. Her reply left me queasy.

"What kind of concerns?"

"Incomplete impact reports, for one. We'll have a sit-down discussion with HR to discuss it further. You can have a union rep there, if you want."

There had been a couple of recent bumps, but Katherine had supervised me for more than three years, and we worked well together. Her formal hardline measure stunned me. And after drafting numerous grant proposals and reports for the program managers, I thought they would bring their concerns directly to me.

Something weird is going on, I thought. *First the meeting last month where Katherine questioned my memory capacity. Now this.*

Angry alarms blared in my head.

When the meeting ended, I was grateful it was nearly five— I was too demoralized to accomplish anything. As I rode the subway home, I analyzed recent reports I'd written for my colleagues and speculated about their possible perceived deficiencies. I came up short.

By the time I reached my stop, I was sure Katherine's sucker punch to my professional credibility had nothing to do with my skills and everything to do with what happened the previous June.

I checked my cellphone contact list to confirm the union representative's info.

The Medusa Warrior

June 14, 2005

I was at my desk, June sun streaming through my Boston office window when I felt telltale fluttering in my stomach. Her back to me, my coworker Fiona sat at her desk. She knew I had epilepsy, and I could have told her what was going on, but in that split second, I hid what was happening as I usually did. *This might pass,* I reasoned. I was in a complex partial seizure's grasp, internal gut prickles spreading from my belly to my face. *Flee the moment and the internal chaos. Take a bathroom break and wait it out.*

I left the office before Fiona noticed anything amiss.

My brain's misfiring neurons triggered the gut prickles, and I was in the throes of a partial seizure, possibly on the brink of losing awareness. Ahead of me I saw the open office area buzzing with people on phones, chairs rasping on linoleum.

If I can just navigate the office one step at a time, and make my way to the bathroom— There, I'd have time to collect myself. I'd been on this brink before and come back. I'd even gone over the awareness cliff and recovered countless times. *I can do this—just get to a private, quiet space!*

I stumbled forward but could only walk about fifteen feet. The flutters in my tummy and tingling on my lips had intensified, my mouth twitching uncontrollably.

What was this? I could usually find my way on autopilot during a seizure. That one overtook me so quickly, there was no way to escape its grip. I cried out involuntarily—then I was oblivious.

Eventually I would hear the following account from my friend and colleague Robin. She said that moaning, I'd walked in circles in the office, my tongue clicking against the top of my mouth like an automatic switch gone haywire. My coworkers tried to restrain me, but even in deeper seizure-haze I just wanted to escape. My limbs jerked and stiffened as I aimlessly paced, saliva frothing from my mouth. My spasming diaphragm pushed air out of my lungs in loud wails.

I woke up en route to New England Medical Center with a walloping headache rivaled by a heavy sensation in my gut as though I'd been hit. But, no. Dread and disappointment gathered in my belly like a lead ball. I'd had a seizure at work, a seizure alarming enough that my colleagues called an ambulance.

I was accustomed to having what are known as complex partial seizures. They typically began with a sense of impending doom followed by brief loss of awareness and, often, some lip smacking. The seizure I'd just had at work was much bigger—a grand mal. I hadn't had a grand mal in ten years, and it blindsided me. Even more upsetting than the seizure's sudden acuteness were the circumstances. Before that day, when I had the occasional seizure at the office, I picked up wherever I left off shortly after it ended. Sometimes the seizures were so small, nobody even noticed them, but even with obvious seizures, I could carry on with my work. That day, however, my colleagues felt compelled to call 911.

I was embarrassed that they'd seen me so vulnerable and incapacitated. Many of them already knew of my epilepsy. That day, ambulance sirens had announced my condition to the whole building. I shuddered at the thought as the medics transferred me to the ER. I wanted to be known as Laura, the grant writer with the tight curly hair, not Laura, the one who has epilepsy.

Her hands deftly wrapping the blue band around my arm to check blood pressure, a nurse took my vitals. "How are you feeling?"

"A little dizzy—my head hurts."

"Yes. They gave you some extra anticonvulsants to stop the seizure. The dizziness will decrease as they wear off."

That's great, but it doesn't help me now. The hospital wanted to release me to somebody, so I called Mark. Although we'd dated only for about six months, we were serious—in fact, we had plans to move in together later that week. Mark had seen me have complex partial seizures.

"This one was definitely a bigger seizure than usual, so my coworkers called 911. But I'm basically okay now," I explained.

"I'm sorry—that sounds awful. Glad you're okay, though."

While I didn't enjoy recounting the horrible story, I knew Mark could handle it. The situation would have scared some boyfriends, but not him.

"I can meet you at the hospital after work," he said.

I spent the long afternoon staring impatiently at the television, stewing about my erratic seizure history. *Why a grand mal today? Was this the beginning of something? Would I have another? Perhaps it was due to excitement about my upcoming move? Who knows?* It wasn't the first time my brain had bowled me over out of the blue. The last grand mal I'd had in 1995 was the first one in fifteen years, and it had prompted my then-neurologist to suggest brain surgery.

"You've tried several medications without success, and this was a bigger seizure. The neurosurgeons would consider you an excellent candidate," he'd said, his face creased with concern. I remember thinking that Dr. H's soft-spoken demeanor and use of the word "excellent" were incompatible with his terrifying surgery proposition.

"Uh, I'd rather just keep the grand mals under control," I'd said after a moment. "You know, go for improved seizure control using additional medication, and skip the surgery." If medication could limit the seizure activity to complex partials, I could manage them. Sure, the seizures I experienced about six times each month were a nuisance, but that paled in comparison to the vision of a scalpel cutting my head open.

Ten years later, as I lay in the hospital bed, the seizure's aftereffects subsiding, I was frustrated. Once a seizure runs its course, a person just needs lots of rest. There's no advantage to being in the hospital. *What a colossal waste of time and resources. I could have recovered just as well at home.* But with my brain temporarily out of control and my colleagues compelled to call 911, I'd lost control of the day. Shortly before I expected Mark to arrive, Fiona came in bearing a modest bouquet.

"Here—these are from everybody in Development," she said, handing me the flowers. Equal rushes of gratitude and embarrassment washed over me.

"How are you feeling?" Fiona's brow furrowed with worry, and I was touched.

"My head hurts a bit, but I'm basically okay." Hoping the slight elevation would demonstrate the truth of my words, I propped my upper body onto my elbows. Compared to how I'd felt during the brain hijack at work, I was flying high. But I also felt scared, vulnerable, and exposed lying flat out in my hospital johnny, pondering seizure patterns. "Mark's going to be here soon—I can't wait to go home. I might have been better off had I'd just gone straight there instead of here."

"This seizure seemed bigger than usual. We were so worried about you." Fiona pushed her curls away from her face and over her wrinkled brow. Her hair had frizzed from the day's humidity.

"Yeah, I understand." Although it distressed me to have wound up in the ER, I didn't blame my colleagues for sending me there. "Thanks for the flowers. I might use a sick day tomorrow, but you can tell everybody I'm fine."

Less than half an hour after Fiona left, I was relieved to see Mark's familiar stocky figure appear in my sterile hospital room. Slightly sweaty from the effort of hauling his workbag across town, he'd come as promised straight from his office. The sun streamed in and glinted off Mark's brown eyes, transforming them to a greenish hazel color. He smiled, his wide grin lighting up his face.

"How are you feeling?" he asked, sitting on the edge of the hospital bed.

"I'm ready to go home."

❧ ❧

I got to the office early on Thursday and threw myself into writing proposals and impact reports coming due, tracking them for our team. My timely arrival strategy worked, as I didn't run into anybody until Fiona got there.

"Hey, there. How are you feeling?"

I longed for basic small talk, but I knew I needed to have an uncomfortable conversation. "I'm fine. I was fine by the time I got

6

home from the hospital. Just a little rattled from the shock of it. The doctor changed my medications. Hopefully that keeps the bigger seizures away. Did others ask after me?"

"I gave Katherine and the other managers an update from the hospital visit. They may have shared that with their teams."

Over the years, Fiona had proven a reliable ally in the face of my seizures. The first time I'd had one in her presence years earlier, I immediately sought refuge in the bathroom until it passed. A little foggy but functional, I returned to our office. That day, I dreaded the conversation I was about to have with Fiona. But the challenge of discussing my epilepsy with Fiona would be relatively small on my confession-spectrum scale—she had enough equanimity and sympathy to hear me out and respond appropriately.

"Is there anything I can do to help if I see you having a seizure?" Fiona had asked.

I was moved by the genuine concern coming from her blue eyes. "Remind me I'm going to be okay. I'm always too panicked during a seizure to remember that."

The rest of my work day was uneventful with nobody asking me about the grand mal. I suspected it partly due to Fiona's staff update, and I was grateful to her.

❧ ❦

Mark and I moved in together as planned the following weekend. We'd met six months earlier through a personal ad I'd placed in the weekly arts newspaper.

I would rather have dated somebody longer before shacking up, but we were both nearing forty. I'd been dating since my twenties and had my share of unsuccessful long- and short-term relationships. Given my experience and the fact that my parents had been married and divorced twice each, I had clear ideas about what I was looking for: a kind, stable partner who also wanted to have a family. And from what I could tell, Mark might fit the bill. We were both on the marriage-and-family fast track. So. when I learned from my dear friends Joyce and Richard that they had a vacant two-bedroom unit on the first floor of their house, I wanted to take it. I was both excited and nervous as I shared the details at dinner the same night. What if Mark thought it was too soon?

"That's great!" Mark exclaimed. We feasted on enchiladas at Rudy's, a local Mexican restaurant. Despite the dim lighting, I could see his joyful smile. Relieved to hear his excitement, I still needed to voice the obvious.

"I know it's kind of fast to live together. But I'm ready to try, and I think the apartment will be a good situation."

"Yes, it's quick, but I want to do it too." Mark reached across the table and put his hand on mine. "When is the unit available?"

Oh, yay. I squeezed his hand.

❧ ☙

Most days leading up to the move, I woke up at dawn. The summer sky lightened obscenely early, shortly after four. I was also excited about moving in with Mark and anxious about the grand mal seizure. What if I had another one?

Mark had lived alone in Boston's South End, and I roomed with two others in a North Cambridge three-bedroom apartment. We hired movers. By late Saturday afternoon, we had officially moved into the Somerville apartment, our mismatched, newly co-owned furniture in place and packed boxes strewn about the unit. About a week after moving in, I woke to the sight of bare walls and unpacked boxes in the middle of the room. The room was a mess, but the mattress felt solid beneath me. His gentle snores breaking the morning silence, Mark slept next to me, I touched Mark's shoulder and found it, too, solid to the touch. He faintly stirred, then went back to his snoring. Relief and tenderness washed over me. We had taken the leap to that messy bedroom and firmly landed. The summer's brightest nights were still in front of us.

"I wonder if I had that big seizure partly because I was excited about our moving in together,' I mused aloud as we got ready for work. "I mean, I am happy about it, but moving is always chaotic. Even happy tumult can bring on seizures."

"I'd rather you not have that negative association with moving in together," Mark said, looking a little miffed.

"Don't worry—I know we did the right thing." Neurological disorders are mysterious. But even if somebody could authenticate a definite cause and effect, I knew I made the right choice.

8

I got a sense of Mark's steadfastness early on, as he didn't run the other way when he first learned I had epilepsy. He didn't freak out. Like Fiona, he asked what he should do if he saw me having a seizure.

I told him to comfort me in the moment. It was only fair to prepare him, so I described what the outward warning signs of a seizure looked like. Of course, I dreaded that inevitable first seizure in Mark's presence. The image of myself seizing in front of Mark embarrassed me. Uncontrollable vulnerability in front of a new friend—no matter how caring—is a humiliating experience. I was also worried that witnessing my seizure would be so scary for Mark, he'd flee. But when the unavoidable moment came three months after we met, I tried to push him away.

Mark and I biked the slushy Minuteman Trail in neighboring Arlington on an early spring day. I was happy to be out in the sun, and undeterred by the messy riding conditions. I plowed ahead into the slush until the familiar twinge in my belly put the kibosh on my ride. *Oh, crap*, I thought, as I pulled over to the side of the trail.

"I'm having a seizure. I have to stop," I called out, bracing the bicycle between my legs as the tummy twinge expanded into full blown tingling across my face.

Mark pulled up next to me. Ugh—I didn't want him to see me in that state. Then I went over my consciousness cliff.

When I came out of the seizure minutes later, Mark stood by my side. I wanted to get as far away from him as possible. The bicycle lay on the path at my feet, and I was tempted to hop on it. I wanted to pump the pedals as hard as I could away from Mark, but in my post-seizure haze, I knew that was impractical, and not the nicest way to end a date.

"How you doing?" Mark asked, placing his hand on my shoulder. Vulnerable to the point of humiliation, I wanted to scream *I can't stand that you're seeing me incapacitated! Leave me alone*! But I knew it irrational to displace anger at my brain onto Mark.

"Fine," I replied. Slush had soaked through my leggings, leaving my shins and thighs damp and chilly. I was exposed in every way.

Later, Mark told me that during the seizure, I'd shoved him back. When he came toward me attempting to help and I warded him off, he feared passersby thought he was harming me.

Mark had the tenacity to see me through the seizure and its accompanying emotional fallout. Once I knew he could withstand both, he'd passed important tests. In the months that followed, I had other seizures while we were together. By then, I felt at peace with his seeing me so exposed, and comfortable accepting his help.

❧ ☙

A month after I landed in the ER, I was scheduled for a midyear evaluation from my manager, Katherine. Katherine was at least twelve years older than I. She never went by Kate or Kathy, and her formal name choice matched her cool, aloof manner. While I appreciated warmth in a supervisor, I could get by without it. I valued Katherine's clear directives and feedback and respected her rejection of traditional female beauty molds. Katherine handed over the evaluation form as she spoke.

"Some of your recent proposals indicate you're not grasping the design and rationale of the programs," she said. "You need to outline those more clearly."

I felt confident about my work going into the meeting, so her words hit like a curveball. I skimmed the evaluation document with relief and noted she checked the "making progress toward meeting objectives" box not the "not meeting objectives" option.

"I will closely review the programs' materials and keep them in mind going forward," I assured Katherine, eager to address any perceived shortcomings. But the meeting launched a two-year mixed message campaign. The timing of Katherine's concerns, so close to the grand mal seizure I'd had at work, set off alarms. I suspected they were related.

In the months following, I took proactive steps to address the issues Katherine raised, and a few months later in November, I received my third-year annual review. That time, Katherine thanked me for my hard work. She noted the impressive amount of fundraising I'd done over the past year. The positive feedback thrilled me, as it allayed my fears. I'd met my goals, gotten my raise, and, most importantly, my boss was happy with my work. Everything was on track.

During the winter, Katherine suggested I change the focus on my fundraising efforts and reach out to corporate donors instead of foundations. We met several times in her office, the small white table between us, her brown trench coat hanging from a hook. Excited to craft a plan and expand my professional skills, I took copious notes. We developed a time frame with next steps, and I was pleased to see a strategy taking shape. I assumed the momentum was a sign that bumps in the road were behind me, but my theory got invalidated a few weeks later. We discussed the initial phase of the corporate outreach plan, and then Katherine switched topics.

"Laura, do you think your seizures affect your memory?" she asked. The loaded inquiry seemed incongruous, given her expressionless face.

Whoa! How did we get from talking about new job responsibilities to my epilepsy?

I took in Katherine's familiar presence for a moment—her calm demeanor, practical short hair style, and sensible navy pantsuit. She emanated the usual down-to-earth, reliable presence, but what a weird question. I felt uncomfortable as if wearing a sleeveless dress on a warm night and a sudden cool breeze raised goosebumps on my skin.

Over the years, I'd had a harder time recalling details like movie plots or actors' names. When I saw people out of context, I often couldn't place their names with their faces, but the slip-ups felt minor. And using writers' tools, I did my damnedest to make sure I tracked things closely at work. Given Katherine's recent positive feedback and forward movement on my work responsibilities, I still thought of her as an ally that day. For better or worse, I answered her unnerving question honestly.

"I'm not sure. My doctors can't tell me for certain whether it's the seizures that affect my memory or the medications I take. But it's likely that one of them does. That's why I take so many notes." I pointed to my notebook on the table between us. Katherine's eye landed on the spiral-bound journal with its red cover distended from the used, wrinkled pages. I smiled weakly. My comprehensive notes proved I was meticulous, but they might not be enough.

"Yes, I guess you do," Katherine observed. She glanced out the window perhaps to distract herself from the uneasy conversation.

"Try to get me a draft of that proposal by the end of the week," she said, as she stood up. The meeting ended, but the exchange triggered more red flags.

Confirming my fears, Katherine issued the formal complaint a month later. As I walked home from the subway that day, I left a phone message for the union representative Carl asking for his help at the meeting with HR the following month.

That night, I railed at Mark over dinner. We sat across from each other at the dining room table, the home-cooked meal laid out before us. I hadn't touched my plate of pesto pasta because I was too busy grousing. "Katherine complained I didn't participate in meetings and my reports were incomplete. That's bullshit! Her November evaluation implied just the opposite. I'm sure it's related to my epilepsy."

"I'm sorry," Mark said. He picked up his fresh bottle of Heineken and tipped it my way. "Want the first sip?" Mark asked. He wanted to mollify me with his characteristic sweet offer, but I wasn't ready.

"No, thanks." I said glumly.

"You can always leave MEDUSA. With all your experience, I'm sure you'd find something else pretty quickly."

"You're right, I could. But this is discrimination. It's wrong—not to mention illegal."

"Yes, but if staying there makes you miserable, is it worth the fight?" Mark reached over and rested his hand on my shoulder. "Just think about it." Mark tried to be helpful, but he didn't understand I considered Katherine's disciplinary action a personal attack I had to fight tooth and nail.

Mark was right about one thing—with my solid background, finding a new job was a viable option. I suspected Katherine and her manager Tracie expected me to do that.

In Greek mythology, a winged human female monster Medusa has venomous snakes for hair. When people looked at her, they supposedly turned to stone because of her ugly fierceness. Perhaps MEDUSA management assumed their negative feedback would immobilize me, and I'd retreat. They didn't know that, while my curly hair wasn't poisonous, when I was a child, that unique attribute resulted in merciless teasing from peers that shaped me into a warrior of sorts.

Katherine and Tracie thought they could scare me away with their undermining and false allegations, but they had another thing coming.

Activist Cultivation

Starting in the late seventies, it was my father who taught me to speak out when I saw something unfair or unjust. My parents divorced when I was four. I lived with my mother in the Bronx.

When I was ten, Dad lived with his second wife in the rural central Massachusetts town of Royalston near the New Hampshire border and participated in activism with local community members. They participated with the widespread Clamshell Alliance to protest against construction of the Seabrook Nuclear Power Plant in Seabrook, New Hampshire. The Town of Royalston voted four times against its construction. Dad hosted meetings of local Clamshell Alliance members the previous year.

Dad's descriptions of the thousands of people at the Seabrook protests and how their actions hindered the power plant's construction uplifted me with the power of the people. I eagerly wanted to contribute in some way.

During that time, a week after visiting my father, I attended a crafts activity at the local library near my Bronx apartment. We made plaster of Paris casts. I loved the simplicity of the task. We mixed water, white powder plaster, and glue. We let it dry for a while, and voila. I had a ready-to-paint piece of art. Dad's Seabrook sit-in stories so inspired me that I made a bright yellow disk and painted the words NO NUKES in neon orange capital letters— yellow for the sun, orange words for the cause.

Shortly before I started eighth grade, Dad's marriage to my younger half brother's mother, Mary, ended, and he moved from Royalston to nearby Wendell. Around the same time, Mom abruptly chose to move our family from the Bronx to suburban Atlanta. I attended two months of eighth grade in Clarkston, Georgia.

When my nine-year-old sister Greta and I flew to visit our father for the holiday break, I decided to move in with Dad. I hadn't planned on moving to Massachusetts, but when Dad invited me, I said yes because I didn't like my stepfather, Geoffrey, and I found the culture shock of living in Georgia too big.

"You're staying here?" Greta demanded when our dad announced it at breakfast during vacation. Worry creases settled on her forehead as guilt pangs wrenched my gut.

"Yes." I spoke softly. "I don't want to live with Geoffrey anymore, and I have more friends here."

"You could stay, too," Dad suggested to Greta.

"No, no. I don't want to do that. Does Mom know yet?" Greta asked me.

"No. I still have to tell her." My body tensed at the thought.

"You should call her today," Dad said. "The sooner she knows, the better." *Easy for him to say*. But I knew he was right—it would be best to get that conversation over.

Later that day I found the rotary phone on the kitchen wall and made the hardest phone call of my life. Dread and guilt welled inside me as I made small talk with her about our trip. I clenched the phone in my hand, squeezed my eyes tight, and redirected the conversation.

"Mom, I've decided to stay here and live at Dad's. I'm not coming back to Georgia with Greta on Monday."

"What? But, why?"

"I want to try living with Dad for a while. I don't have any friends in Georgia. I know some kids here–I think I'll be happier." I didn't mention the longstanding tensions with Geoffrey, –a sore spot she already knew about.

"Oh." I heard the pain in her voice. "What about Greta? Is your father sending Greta home?"

"Yes, she'll be on the plane Monday."

I was relieved when she asked to speak with Dad and thankful to escape her resentment and distress. But Mom's anger resulted in several months' silent treatment. Looking back, I know moving in with Dad proved a good choice for me, but at the time, I'd unintentionally divorced my mother and sister in the process. The move put almost a thousand miles and immeasurable emotional distance between me and my mother. The latter was never completely bridged.

With the backdrop of that familial turmoil, it came as no shock that I had a grand mal seizure about two weeks after moving in with Dad. I'd had one six months earlier—the first in seven years—and my doctors had said it likely occurred due to hormonal shifts related to puberty.

My father enrolled me at the local high school, Mahar Regional in Orange, and I was just beginning to find my footing with the new routine.

One afternoon, I invited my friend Peter over after school. I was buddies with his sister, Lorien. When I visited the previous summer, they were both part of my larger Wendell posse. We spent the days biking hilly dirt roads, rambling through woods, and swimming in Gridley's Pond where locals often skinny-dipped. Peter and I had some classes together. I found Mahar's eighth-grade curriculum easier than at my school in the Bronx, so what I considered undemanding academics allowed for interspersing homework with goofing off.

Dad got home and found the two of us sprawled in the living room, our notebooks open and unused, Pink Floyd's "Another Brick in The Wall" blasted on the stereo. Peter was wearing a blue sweatshirt, the sleeves intentionally ripped in the style of the *Warriors* movie characters.

"Getting the homework done, huh?" Dad asked, a sarcastic smile crossing his face. "Peter, what's with the ripped clothes? You going for the punk effect? The raggedy attire isn't exactly fetching."

Peter rolled his eyes.

"Oh, whatever, Stan. This is how everybody's dressing."

Dad shrugged back.

"Whatever," he agreed. "I'm making some split pea soup, if you're interested," he offered.

"Nah, my mom is picking me up in about a half hour on her way home."

I relaxed in the living room as I basked in their chitchat. Their rapport was symbolic—it was my new home, I was settling in, I had friends and family around me.

Then I felt the telltale creeping sensation in the pit of my stomach. *Oh no. A friggin' seizure is about to ruin everything!* Peter had witnessed my seizures before, but when I felt the tingling, I needed to get away. *Maybe I can wait the seizure out in the kitchen and then rejoin Peter before he leaves.*

"Um, I'll be right back," I said, leaving the room. My voice sounded normal, but as I walked toward the kitchen, the prickling in my belly had spread to my face, and my tongue was clicking uncontrollably against the roof of my mouth. Dad looked up from the stove.

"Laura! Are you okay?" The last thing I remember was panic flashing across Dad's face as he dashed toward me.

❧ ☙

I woke up disoriented in my own bed. My digital clock said 2:37, and it was pitch black, so I knew it was the middle of the night. I tried to recount my last conscious moments, but my throbbing head interfered and triggered an involuntary moan.

"Laura, you're up. How are you feeling?" I heard Dad's voice—he had set up camp in the far corner of my room. I pulled the metal cord on the ceiling light over my bed. Dad sat bleary-eyed on the ottoman, his back against the wall, the felt white cushion sagging beneath him. "You had a seizure—a big one."

"Yeah, I know. I think it was a grand mal," I said, recalling the one I'd had at school six months earlier. *Thank goodness I am home this time.* "Did Peter see it?"

"Just the beginning. Katie came by pretty soon after the seizure started." *Just as well.* Though I trusted Peter to keep it to himself, the less he saw the better. *But what if it happened again when I was at school? Then all my new classmates would know!*

"Did we go to a hospital?" I was confused. Could I really have slept through an entire hospital visit?

"No. The nearest hospital is fifteen miles away, and the roads are slippery. I decided it was safer to stay home and see how you were doing when you woke up."

At the time, I was relieved to be home and happy about Dad's choice. Years later, I realized what a tough decision my father had made that night. He'd witnessed many partial seizures but hadn't seen me have a grand mal for six years. In his shoes, I might have been too scared to take a wait-and-see-approach if my daughter was seizing. But Dad was very analytical by nature, and we lived in the middle of nowhere where the nearest hospitals had minimal staff and amenities. I imagine he did a quick, informal cost-benefit analysis of Athol Memorial Hospital's potential care level versus the treacherous drive and concluded it safer to stay home.

When I woke up late the next morning, a coating of snow blanketed the world outside.

"No school today—they declared it a snow day," Dad announced. Relief washed over me as I watched flakes propelled by the wind and haphazardly swirling over the lawn. Nobody would miss me while I recovered. By the next day I'd be fine to go back to school, and I was pretty sure Peter wouldn't tell our classmates what happened.

❧ ☙

Mahar Regional High provided a hands-on education in regionalization's effects on rural school districts. In New York City, the district parses the children into schools typically named after a neighborhood or person but primarily known by its impersonal number. In rural areas like Wendell, school districts bundle children from neighboring towns into one large regional facility. Mahar had kids from New Salem, Wendell, Orange, and Petersham. They had previously attended their local elementary schools. I was too naive to realize it, but there were significant differences in the towns' residents. Demographically similar with largely Caucasian populations, each of the smaller towns had a mix of agrarian families, wealthy families thanks to trust funds or other inheritance, or working class families. With larger Orange primarily working class, I soon saw the communities as culturally diverse and worlds apart politically .

I'd spent the previous summer in Wendell, so I was socially cushioned by my local buddies and the town's alternative culture and I didn't feel the need to integrate fully at Mahar. Just like in Georgia, at school I was the new kid with the wild curls secretly hoping I wouldn't have another big seizure at school. I kept up my studious tendencies. Other than seeking out my Wendell friends in the cafeteria and during classes, I kept to myself in the hallways between periods, a loner checking in with my locker. Discreetly blending in was an enviable unattainable prospect thanks to my curly hair and New York accent.

At Mahar, I didn't care as much, partly because after moving twice in three months, I learned every school had jerks not worth trying to win over. But my Wendell friends fueled my indifference, and I hung out with them after school. Influenced by our families and a Wendell hippie enclave, we talked about political issues. Questioning feminine conventions was a favorite of mine and my girlfriends, Lorien, Ellen, and Grace. Such questioning was easy to do—even encouraged—in Wendell, where none of the adults I knew had typical day jobs, and the women didn't wear makeup or high heels and dresses.

I eagerly threw myself into the town's counterculture and began viewing the world through an inquisitional lens. As I probed, I decided there were more important things in life than fitting in at school. During those months at Mahar Regional, my new outlook led to my own mini protest. Long before Colin Kaepernick was born, my Wendell friends and I had discussed how disingenuous we thought the Pledge of Allegiance.

"'One nation under God with liberty and justice for all?' That's bogus," Lorien said.

"Yeah, it should say 'one nation divided into many, with liberty and justice for rich white men,'" I replied. Every day, the principal said the Pledge of Allegiance over the loudspeaker, and all the students and staff stood to recite it. After the discussion with Lorien, I didn't want to do it. I already didn't say it—a lot of people didn't— but mere silence was vague. Sitting down during the principal's recitation would be an unambiguous statement. Yet I'd be drawing negative attention to myself at school, which made me anxious.

I mentioned my possible plan to Dad over dinner one February night, and his response buoyed my determination. "You have every right to sit during the pledge. I don't blame you for choosing to sit it out—I think it's a great idea."

I decided to put my plan into action the next morning.

Homeroom was abuzz with my classmates' morning banter and smelled like wet woolens. When the daily ceremonial beep honked through the loudspeaker signaling the principal's announcements, my body was rigid with anxiety. I willed myself to stay seated and folded my hands under my chin. I kept my gaze on my desk as the pledge's words floated through the air. I looked up as it ended, registered my classmates' indifference, and Mr. Torstensen's agitated gaze fixed on me. I wasn't surprised when he called me to his desk as the bell rang. While I expected the ensuing exchange and silently cheered my accomplishment, my heart rate picked up as I approached his desk.

"Yes, what did you want, Mr. Torstensen?" I asked, feigning ignorance.

Mr. Torstensen was in his fifties and seemed extremely tall to me.

"I noticed you didn't stand up for the Pledge of Allegiance this morning."

"That's right. I don't believe in what it stands for, so I don't think I should have to stand up for it." I'd memorized the words in advance, so they flowed out of my mouth.

"You have to stand up for the pledge—I can't have you disrupting homeroom like this."

"But Mr. Torstensen, if I don't believe in something, you can't force me to stand up—I don't think that's allowed." My nerves were rattled, but I held my ground. When Mr. Torstensen cleared his throat, I knew I had won.

"Well, we'll see what Mr. Edminister has to say. You're dismissed," he said, referring to the principal..

Sweat dripped down my sides as I exited the classroom, but inside I smiled. I had made it over the first hurdle. I knew I'd have to speak with the principal, but at that moment I didn't care. I was exhilarated that I had stood up —or sat down —for my apparently controversial belief.

The next morning, Mr. Torstensen sent me directly to the principal's office. "They're waiting for you down there," he said without malice. But the words sounded threatening, as though Mr. Edminister and his colleagues were anticipating my arrival with big scary plans like detentions.

When I got to the office, I met with the Assistant Principal, Mr. Hargraves, who ushered me into his office and guided me to the chair across from his desk. He wrinkled his nose and placed a forefinger along its side. At first, I thought he had to sneeze. Then I gathered he was probably nervous and, like Mr. Torstensen, he didn't really want to have the conversation. The realization empowered me. Mr. Hargraves proposed I spend homeroom in the library.

"When you arrive, you will check in with Mr. Torstensen and let him know that you're here. Then I would like you to go to the library during homeroom. Is that okay with you?"

I thought for a moment. *I might feel isolated in the library, and the other kids would surely notice my absence. I would not be blending in. Would there be any repercussions?* Then I recalled the conversation I had with Dad the other night—it was a great idea, he'd said. Dad's words and Mr. Hargraves's uneasiness galvanized me. I was taking a stand for what I believed in, and Mr. Hargraves was accommodating it.

"Yes, sir. That's fine." Mr. Hargraves looked relieved.

"Good. We'll start this routine tomorrow. I'll tell the librarian to expect you." *It seemed like everybody was expecting me.* I left for my next class.

The librarian was happy to host me for homeroom, but my schoolmates were not as accepting of the irregularity. Getting banished from homeroom was big news at Mahar Regional, and it spread through the school like wildfire. By the end of the week, some kids hurled insults at me.

"Communist!" a boy several grades above me hissed as he passed me in the hall. I'd never seen him before. Was he talking to me? When the same intended indignity got tossed my way by others two more times while I went through the hall to algebra class, clearly they meant it to intimidate me. A small part of me enjoyed the negative attention as it reinforced that I'd stood up for what I believed in. But isolation mitigated my elation, as I was the only person on the crusade. Even my Wendell buddies stayed on the sidelines as I dealt with the aftermath.

While my friends' inaction disappointed me, it didn't surprise me or even make me resentful. I understood the value of obscurity. After checking in with Mr. Torstensen, I went to the library for homeroom and read to myself. When I felt alone, I reminded myself that I didn't need friendships from insult-hurling copycats. I could see my real friends outside of school.

The impulse to stand up for what was fair compelled me to join community activist groups during college and beyond. I sought out UMass, Amherst political organizations often housed in jam-packed dingy offices furnished with messy desks and old couches and lit by bright fluorescent, rod-shaped bulbs. I attended weekly meetings of the Western Mass Latin America Solidarity Committee, where I sat on grubby furniture to plan protests to oppose U.S. policies in Central America. I distributed fliers and made phone calls to help spread the word. I loved collaborating with others and organizing to impact the world around me, a passion I developed watching my father.

When I dealt with MEDUSA's response to my grand mal seizure, I turned to my father for advice. He suggested helpful strategies for pushing back, and although the advice wasn't easy, it was effective.

❧ ☙

Eight months after I moved in with my father, I completed eighth grade at Mahar Regional in Orange, and he moved us to New Jersey. Adjusting to a new school is always hard, but acclimating with the threat of having a seizure lurking presented an additional challenge. In fact, having seizures in school sucked even when you weren't the new kid.

During adolescence, my seizures increased in severity and number. Inevitably I had some at school in front of my teachers and classmates. The first time it happened, I was thirteen in seventh grade, and I still lived in the Bronx with my mother. Like any teen, I wanted to get by and blend in, but the seizure uptick made that a tall order.

New York City middle schools include grades seven through nine. I loved starting junior high school because it felt like a level playing field. Everybody aged into the school at the same time, so there wasn't a preestablished social hierarchy. As I navigated seventh grade, I wasn't part of the in-crowd, but I had a reputation for being smart and reliable. By June, I'd made it through the year without having noticeable seizure activity at school—just an occasional absence seizure that only I could detect. Most of my schoolmates didn't even know I had epilepsy, and those from my elementary school cohort had likely forgotten.

Two weeks prior to summer break, en route to English class, I felt a queasy sensation in my stomach. I knew it was a seizure, but it had been so long since I'd had one, I was flabbergasted. *What's going on? Who's going to see this?* Suddenly an adult I didn't recognize approached me, held her hand before my face, and asked me how many fingers she was holding up. Then I lost my grip on the world. I woke up in Jacobi Hospital in the Bronx with a splitting headache. Resurfacing from the seizure felt like a mental swim through a junkyard full of jagged discarded metal objects, so I didn't immediately notice the nurse hovering nearby.

"You had a seizure—a big one. They called your mother. She's on her way," she informed me. I hadn't had a grand mal for almost six years! Geez. Nothing was more embarrassing than being publicly clobbered by my brain chaos at school. I'd done such a good job keeping my epilepsy off my classmates' radar. *Who knows what they saw? Uncontrollable twitching? Did I pee my pants at school? Ugh!*

My mother picked me up at Jacobi, and I slept off the side effects of the seizure at home. I woke up long after dinner and learned my friends had stopped by to see if I was okay. I was disappointed to miss them but comforted that they'd visited. If my friends were checking on me, they probably weren't going to write me off despite my body's abnormality. I was correct, but my mother abruptly chose to move to Atlanta four months later, so I lost all those friends.

I wound up moving several times before I finished high school. At each new school, I found assimilation challenging due to my curly hair and my epilepsy. After leaving Mahar Regional in Massachusetts, Dad and I moved to New Jersey. I started ninth grade at Cedar Ridge High School in the town of Old Bridge and attended for two years. I decided to stand for the pledge, but as the new kid with the kinky hair in a place where few others had tight curls, I was still conspicuous. Within the first week, the head cheerleader Charlene dubbed me Harpo Marx, so echoes of "Harpo!" followed me in the schoolyard and cafeteria.

I went to school with my reddish-brown curls a shapeless frizzy mass framing my face as I assessed the social landscape. Cedar Ridge High was the fourth school I'd attended in twelve months, so I had intuitive sensibilities about whom to seek out and whom to circumvent. I knew to avoid the belligerent kids who had to demonstrate their dominant status over the class—I was too soft-spoken to fight them off. I wouldn't waste time on the popular cheerleader types—with my hair and lack of makeup, there was no way I'd fit in with them. I didn't want to cheerlead anyway. Mixed in with the trend setters and mean alpha kids, there were always a couple of castoffs. Often watchful and quiet, they offered intelligent insights during class discussions, and they didn't join when mean kids threw their weight at vulnerable kids like me.

Within a couple weeks, I befriended Marcy. Marcy was Jewish and had also lived in the Bronx, two commonalities that drew us together. She kept to herself, and her wardrobe consisted of practical clothes including plaid shirts and plain cable-knit sweaters—definitely no cool Jordache jeans. I could tell that, like my Wendell friends, she had an interest in the outside world. Three weeks into the school year, I sat down across from her in the cafeteria at lunch time.

"We're going to be friends," I announced, as we dug into our respective trays. My definitive statement hung between us as the scent of flavorless chicken patties wafted in the air. My awkward declaration was spot on. Marcy's hair was also somewhat curly, and her tresses were imperfectly coiffed, flat on top, bushy on the bottom. A couple weeks later, I confided to her about my epilepsy.

"The seizures usually only last a couple minutes," I explained. "I don't need to go to the doctor."

"Is there anything somebody should do to help you?"

"The best thing is to walk me to the nurse's office or a quiet place to recover in private." I had yet to have a seizure at that school, but it was only a matter of time before classmates would see me at the mercy of misfiring neurons. With my social status already low, I knew when my classmates witnessed a seizure that my rank would sink further. I coped with the inevitability by ignoring my anxiety over it.

My Cedar Ridge epilepsy outing took place a couple of months later during gym class. I was playing tennis with Marcy. As I whacked the ball, I felt the tingling sensations in my belly. *Oh, no. Here it comes, right in the middle of gym class, no less.* I took stock of the room and saw Charlene and her buddies laughing together in the bleachers. Then my tongue uncontrollably clicked against the roof of my mouth as my right arm went slack. *Thank goodness Marcy is here.* She'd seen me have a seizure after school. She would know what was going on and explain to the others.

"I'm having a seizure," I told Marcy, panic waves rising from my stomach, and spreading across my face. I was more alarmed by the setting than the seizure. Keeping on top of the tennis ball, proving myself a decent player—or at least not incompetent—to a gymnasium full of boisterous classmates — offered enough challenge. On top of it, my brain was in turmoil.

I blanked out as Marcy walked toward my side of the net.

Later, Marcy told me that our gym teacher Mrs. Ferguson freaked out, put the kibosh on the others' tennis games, and circled around me like a headless chicken. While everybody watched, she demanded somebody get the principal, nurse, and an ambulance. I imagine the combination of a seizing student and rowdy kids were too much. Looking back, I can even feel some sympathy for Mrs. Ferguson, but at the time, Marcy's account vexed me. Mrs. Ferguson's response only drew more of my peers' attention and made a bigger spectacle of me.

When I came to, I was alone in the nurse's office, the school nurse hovering over me. "Are you okay, Laura?" she asked.

"Yes. I had a seizure, but it's over."

I looked at the clock, and calculated the periods, which took more effort than usual: gym was over, English was underway, and lunch would begin in about a half hour. Wasn't the English teacher, Mr. Nester, giving us a quiz? If I left at the moment, would I have enough time to complete it?

"Can I go back to class?"

"Why don't you stay and relax for a while. Mrs. Ferguson was worried. She wanted Principal Dewey to call an ambulance, but I told her I'd watch you for a while instead. I called your father, and he agreed with this plan."

"I don't need to go to the hospital—I'm fine." And other than feeling foggy, I was. No medical care could treat my crushing combination of shame, humiliation, annoyance, and embarrassment that my classmates had seen me so out of sorts. I felt guilty that my body had caused so much disruption. I just wanted to put the seizure behind me, resume my day, and prove I was back to normal.

"Why don't you relax here until fourth period ends and then join the others?" Nurse Karen suggested.

"Okay," I agreed reluctantly. *So much for Mr. Nester's quiz*, I thought. *I wonder which of my classmates noticed my seizure and exactly what they saw. Hopefully they won't make a big deal at lunch time.*

The bell rang, Nurse Karen granted me permission to leave, and I went to the lunchroom. I scanned the room and determined that Charlene and her posse were in the far corner. I got lunch, spotted Marcy, and sat down across from her. I noticed only a couple of concerned glances from students who were in gym with me, as I walked from the line to Marcy's table.

"I thought they might send you home," Marcy observed.

"No. I'm okay now. How was the English quiz?"

"Oh, you know—Mr. Nester's quizzes are more like tests. There were three long answer essay questions about *Romeo and Juliet*."

"You gotta love Mr. Nester—he sticks it to us, doesn't he?" I was relieved Marcy rolled with my deflection.

Marcy's friendship got me through ninth and tenth grades in New Jersey. Then Dad decided it was time to move again, that time to a Boston suburb called Littleton. I knew Littleton High was going to be tough. There were only about four hundred kids in the whole school, and most of them had known each other since kindergarten. I'd been experimenting with my hair, futilely attempting to shape it with headbands and barrettes, but it was still somewhat formless, especially when humidity frizzed it out. By the end of the first school day, the alpha kids identified themselves.

"Wow, you've got quite got a head of hair," Rob exclaimed. He was tall and broad with straight short black hair—probably a jock. His words were neutral, but based on his grin and the way he projected them to an audience of friends, I recognized the dig.

"Yeah—Laura's got a huge head of hair," Jeffrey chimed in.

The kids comingled the taunting words in their Boston accent, and from that day, I was tagged Hedda by Rob as the other caustic meanies followed suit.

I promptly neutralized my New York accent and identified the quiet castoffs. I found four detectable by their basic hairstyles and unglamorous garb: Moragh, Jessica, Brian, and Michelle. Where the popular kids dressed in trendy, bold-striped shirts, my new friends wore simple button-downs and baggy sweatpants. Michelle's stick-straight brown hair parted in the middle framed her impish smile. Moragh had a unique name, red hair, and an inordinate number of freckles to boot. Jessica's hair had some wave to it, though it didn't hold a candle to my kinky mop.

Unlike me, Jessica had perfected the art of sassy comeback, handy in the school cafeteria where we often had lunch together. One day, Moragh, Brian, Jessica, and Michelle had identical school lunch fare, a precut fried fish square complemented by gooey mayonnaise-drenched coleslaw. I hated fishcakes, so I ate my lunch from home—a simple cheese sandwich, an apple on the side. Rob sauntered up to our table, friends in tow, a menacing grin on his face. My body tensed, and I was grateful Jessica was at the end of the table, physically closer to Rob than I.

"Hey, Hedda, is your lunch betta?" Rob asked. The other boys laughed appreciatively at his poetic quip. That they thought that clever made my eyes roll. The only reason they could concoct so many rhymes with Hedda was because their close-to-Boston accents caused them to drop their Rs. Eventually they would learn my sister's name, and go ballistic with taunts of *Hey, Hedda, where's Greta?* I wanted to tell Rob how dumb his accent sounded, but I was an outnumbered outlier—the only one with home lunch, tight curls, and New York City inflections.

I silently fumed, the hard cafeteria bench digging into my taut backside as Jessica closely watched the exchange. Her light blue button-down shirt had a square pocket over the chest.

"Screw you," she snapped at Rob. Giggling amongst themselves, Rob and his pals ambled to another table. "He's a jerk," Jessica noted, and we all agreed. Maybe she felt a sense of solidarity with me due to the wave in her blondish locks. Perhaps she didn't like Rob. Though Jessica didn't regularly make a point of sticking up for me, starting that day, I trusted her.

When the first seizure happened at Littleton High School, Moragh was nearby. We were in Spanish class, the teacher reviewing future tense verb conjugation. Foreign language came easy to me, so I was only half listening when the creeping seizure sensations began in my belly. *Uh, oh. Here it comes.* I reflexively looked at my wrist, checking the time.

Sometimes it seemed I could ward off the brain chaos if I grounded myself in the moment. The trick wasn't foolproof, though. I panicked when I realized I'd left my watch at home. I desperately needed to figure out the time. I hunched over my desk and fidgeted with my pen. *What time was it? What time was it? I'd be okay if somebody could just tell me the time.* Then I blanked out.

When I emerged from seizure, I spotted Moragh sitting at an adjacent desk, and relief gushed through me.

"What time is it?" I whispered anxiously.

"Five past one," she replied. I grounded myself by ten past although I felt vague and dreamy. I didn't know who else had noticed exactly what I'd done or said. Seemingly indifferent to my seizure the Spanish teacher reviewed a new vocabulary list. Either she was unaware or Moragh had explained it to her. Later, I was embarrassed to learn that I'd repeatedly wailed *What time is it?* out loud to the entire class during the seizure.

Like Marcy in Old Bridge, my friends Moragh and the others sustained me for the two years I attended Littleton High. But what truly got me through my junior and senior years was looking forward to college. Prior to leaving New Jersey, Dad had helped me gather my Cedar Ridge High transcripts. He carefully signed the release forms and reminded me to gather the paperwork before we moved to Massachusetts. I'd stashed them safely away in a manila envelope. I was a solid B+ student, and Dad had made it clear that he would pay for college.

By the time I got to Littleton, I'd traveled through all forty-eight continental states and lived in four of them. No matter how domineering the Littleton alpha mean kids were, I knew those Rs weren't the only way people talked. There would be students from all over the world at college, and some of them would even have hair as curly as mine.

Domestic Developments

Many years after my high school experiences, managing the MEDUSA drama proved miserable, but at least happy transforming milestones peppered my personal life. When we moved in together, I was almost thirty-nine and Mark a year and a half older. We wanted to start a family, so my loudly ticking biological clock played a large role in our decision. We considered living together our test run for marriage.

After years of experience of living with others, I was a pro at rolling with my roommates' sometimes annoying quirks, and I could do the same for Mark. When I discovered he didn't like the top sheet tucked in on the bottom—a *must* for me to consider the bed made—I learned to leave the top sheet loose on his side. During the first year in our Somerville unit, we discovered numerous other minor but manageable grumbles over each other's habits. Most important to me, living with Mark confirmed what I suspected: Mark was kind, reliable, and trustworthy. He wasn't going anywhere despite my seizures or the bedmaking quandary. Within seven months of moving in, we began planning our wedding for the following summer and talking about getting pregnant.

"You know I'm turning forty next fall. There's no time to waste," I said to Mark. We lingered eating waffles and sipping coffee at the breakfast table on a weekend morning. More than anything, the possibility of birth defects related to my age freaked me out, especially since I hoped to have two children.

"Well, I'm a year and a half older—not exactly a spring chicken, either," Mark said. He got up to get more coffee. "Want me to warm your cup?"

I nodded. "All the more reason to move fast," I said. "Of course, your body plays a far smaller role in this."

"True, but I still want to be strong and healthy enough to do things like teaching my kid to bike ride or taking them to soccer practice."

Given our earlier talks, I wasn't surprised by the ease of the conversation. But in addition to worrying about genetic deficiencies due to my age, Mark and I would have to navigate the inevitable challenges due to my epilepsy. I knew it would be tricky, but my desire to parent ran deep. Growing up, I was one of those kids who envisioned being a mom someday while playing with her Baby Drowsy doll. By the time Mark and I sipped coffee that day, the wish felt so keen, I wouldn't let the challenges of my medical condition stop me.

"Assuming I get pregnant, once there's a baby, my seizures will sometimes complicate things." We hadn't discussed the obvious fact. We needed to talk about the elephant in the room.

"I know," he said. Mark's response implicitly acknowledged his willingness to take on the complexities and pleased me. When I imagined having one of my typical seizures while caring for a baby, the seizures seemed surmountable.

"I truly feel like if I was holding a baby or pushing a stroller when a seizure started, I'd have enough warning to put the baby safely in its crib or on the floor or put the brakes on the stroller, stop walking, and wait it out."

He had witnessed many of my seizures by then.

"Yeah, that's probably true. It's not great, though."

"No, it's not," I agreed. "I could try to call you afterward, although by the time I'm able to do that, the seizure would be well behind me."

"I suppose so. I've seen your seizures. I think we'll get through this alright."

Woo hoo! Mark agreed the seizures were manageable. Not everybody would have, but Mark was an optimist by nature. His inherently hopeful outlook complemented my pessimistic tendencies. Over the years, I sometimes found him too optimistic, and we quibbled. But that morning, I was grateful and relieved about his positive viewpoint, as it enabled him to take the leap with me.

"Me, too. We'd better take full advantage of these lazy Saturday mornings. Hopefully, they're numbered," I said.

At my next neurological checkup, I spoke with my then neurologist, Dr. K, about pregnancy. She had taken my case from Dr. H a year earlier, so I was still getting to know her. She seemed warm and personable, but like every neurologist I'd ever had, she had yet to discover my secret seizure-control sauce. She gave the basic neurological exam that included walking heel to toe, following her finger with my eyes, and checking reflexes. I always passed the simple tests with flying colors, but the results had no correlation with seizure control.

"I'm hoping to get pregnant this year," I announced as she tapped my knee with her reflex hammer.

"Okay. We'll have to get you off carbamazepine first, as that can be dangerous for a developing baby. We can replace it with lamotrigine, which has no side effects on the pregnancy."

"Great. Hopefully, it will control the seizures better, too," I said. I'd tried so many medications by then that I wasn't optimistic. "Do others of your patients with seizures like mine hire nannies to help with childcare as a precaution?" I asked. Mark and I had discussed the option and concluded it seemed unnecessary given my seizures' infrequency and recovery time.

"No. My patients who hire nannies do so because they want a break from the work," she said.

"So, you think I'll be able to do this without hired help?"

"You'll have to be especially careful about certain things—like changing the baby on the floor, not a table for example. If you take precautions, you should be okay."

Dr. K outlined a three-month schedule for the medication change. Mark and I would start trying to get pregnant after that.

We were lucky. By our wedding day five months later, the pregnancy was three months along and early enough that I didn't show in my pale pink wedding dress.

When I shared our plan with a few of my closest friends and family members, I was thrilled——I was going to have a family! Most people were excited for me, but when I shared the news with my father by phone, I received a lot of flak.

"You shouldn't be alone with a baby. What happens if you have a seizure? How can you be sure the baby will be safe?"

His agitation didn't surprise me. He'd previously expressed concern about other choices I'd made, like bike riding. Given his logical left-brained nature, there was no way he'd understand the devastation I'd feel if I chose not to have kids.

"I always have a pre-seizure warning—the aura—when I'm still aware. That will give me enough time to put the baby down or stop the stroller or whatever."

"You should hire somebody to stay with you," he said adamantly.

"That would be expensive. Also unnecessary. I talked about hiring a nanny with my neurologist. She agreed I don't need to."

"That's ridiculous. Your doctor's an idiot."

I expected the conversation to be hard, but my father's reproach stung more than I anticipated. His contention that I wouldn't be able to parent well because I had epilepsy viscerally hurt me.

"I understand why you're concerned. I've lived with the seizures all my life. I don't have them that often, and when I do, they're not that big. It's not good, I agree. But I think I recover from them quickly enough that I can handle taking care of my child."

"Well, that sounds insanely dangerous to me."

"Okay, that's you. It's my decision."

The discussion was over.

The obstacles others constructed over my epilepsy left me indignant. First MEDUSA implied that I couldn't do my job well. Then my father implied I couldn't parent well. While my seizures hindered me and caused others panic, I was the expert when it came to their true impact on me. My father's words and MEDUSA's insinuations undermined everything I knew on an intuitive level. They landed like a punch to my gut and weighed me down like a rucksack full of unnecessary goods.

My father and I had multiple iterations of the discussion—some with Mark, some without, some before I was a parent, some years after. They always ended poorly with no resolution and my feelings tattered.

I once had a boyfriend who jokingly called my father "Manly Stanley," referencing his gruff manner built into his DNA. The nickname assuaged my pain a little. I knew Dad's abrasion came from fear and even love. But when Manly Stanley gets an idea in his head about how *he* thinks things should be done, he is unable to see beyond his way. Over the years, he's made it abundantly clear that had he been in my shoes, he wouldn't have had kids. I'm forever glad I didn't take his advice on that choice.

My father was a computer programmer and then a math teacher by profession, and I'd inherited some of Stanley's left-brain tendencies. I understood my father's concerns. I knew seizures and babies presented a challenging combination, but I was up for it, especially after some careful calculating. I would be alone with the baby only while Mark was at work. With Mark gone fifty hours per week, I would be alone with the baby about twenty-six percent of the time. During a typical month when I had ten seizures, I'd have to deal with the situation two or three times. I knew it wasn't ideal and presented some risks. I allayed my fears by reminding myself that I typically recovered quickly. And ninety-nine-plus percent of the time, I wasn't in the throes of a seizure, I would be thoughtful and so, so careful. I had to be to make up for the seizures.

My own childhood was rife with imperfections. My immature parents' marriage lasted five years. Their failed remarriages tossed me in the midst of insecure familial landscapes followed by multiple moves during adolescence. I was certain Mark and I could create a more secure family environment for our child despite my seizures.

The MEDUSA Drama

A few weeks following the March meeting with MEDUSA HR, confirmation of my pregnancy with my first child bolstered my resolve to stay at MEDUSA. The boy was due seven months later in January, and I wanted to take advantage of MEDUSA's generous maternity benefits.

I kicked into high alert mode. I sent my manager Katherine long, detailed memos outlining responses to the concerns she raised and detailing new corporate outreach job responsibilities. I regularly copied Carl, the union rep, and Belinda, the human resources associate. I kept careful notes on every exchange I had with Katherine and other program staff involved with the corporate outreach project.

Given the complexity of my professional life leading up to Liam's birth, an easy pregnancy offered welcome relief from anxiety brought on by Katherine's multiple mixed messages. She did a midyear evaluation in August that noted "poor strategic choices" but acknowledged my "adequate" job performance.

More than the criticisms, I was concerned about the time frame. Katherine based her assessment on the new job description she'd only recently outlined. I hadn't had time to learn and implement it. The insufficient assessment period combined with the unfair evaluation glared since I thought MEDUSA wanted me to leave. I assumed Katherine's critical words and abridged timeframe comprised MEDUSA's strategies to undermine my work.

That fall, I also had an increase in complex partial seizures, many of them at work. It wasn't unusual for me to have three noticeable seizures within a week. In September, I had four seizures within three days in the office where other coworkers had seen them. Three out of four times, only Fiona or others on my small team witnessed them. All mid-sized complex seizures, big enough that others could recognize something wrong with me, but small enough that I could resume working after they passed.

The fourth seizure occurred during a development department meeting attended by fifteen people including Tracie, the department head. My friend Robin escorted me out of the meeting. At the elevator, when I resurfaced from the seizure's murky lava, I protested Robin's decision to chaperone me to my office.

"But what about the staff meeting?" I asked. "I missed the end of Callie's presentation."

"Laura, you need to rest," she said firmly. A ding announcing the elevator's arrival underscored her directive. "Here, let's go." Deep inside I knew Robin was right, so I let her lead me to my empty office. "Will you be okay, if I head back to the meeting?" she asked.

"Yeah, I'll be fine. You can share your notes from the last of Callie's presentation later."

Eager to complete an unfinished impact report, I turned to my computer too drained to focus. The seizure's aftereffects had passed, but the repetition of my circumstances left me exhausted: another seizure at work, another instance where I had to prove myself and assure others. Yes, my seizures confounded others and sometimes scared them.

Later, I heard the elevator's distant ding as people returned from the staff meeting. *Here we go again*, I thought. *Now I'd have to face more coworkers and prove that I am okay, capable, and competent despite my epilepsy.*

I forced myself to concentrate on reports so I wouldn't dwell on what happened in the meeting room. Eventually, I got Robin's account. Apparently, Callie had just rattled off her program achievements the moment I lost awareness, and I let out a large questioning moan that sounded like a response to Callie. Everybody in the room looked my way. My outburst puzzled everyone except for Robin, who had known me for more than fifteen years. On the opposite side of the table from me, she got up and did her best to lead me out of the room toward the elevators. After that meeting, Robin took it upon herself always to sit next to me at our monthly staff meetings. I never asked her to do it nor did we talk about her seating choice, but in retrospect, I am grateful for her thoughtful gesture.

I didn't learn what transpired during that meeting until years later. By then, enough time had passed that I could laugh instead of feeling embarrassed. But on that fall afternoon, my report writing provided a pleasant distraction from thinking about the situation—which I could only imagine—in the meeting room. Working hard also offered the only way I knew how to prove that my epilepsy didn't have to impede my job performance.

In response to the uptick in my seizures, Tracie asked me to speak about my epilepsy at a monthly staff meeting. *Give a quick overview of what a seizure is and what people should do if you have one,* she'd said.

Tracie's request startled me, as it required me to draw attention to my health issues. *Was it even legal?* Although not happy about Tracie's ask, I was adept at playing epilepsy educator, so I knew exactly what I would and wouldn't say. I wouldn't tell them the whole truth—Katherine's negative feedback and raging hormones related to pregnancy likely contributed to seizure increase.

I'd give the basic summary.

Edgy about the task ahead of me, I sat through the October staff meeting with perhaps sixteen people at the table. By then, almost all of them knew I had epilepsy, although I had had frank conversations about it with not more than a third of them. The others and I interacted distantly enough that I hadn't felt compelled to provide explanations until Tracie had the nerve to request public clarification.

When Tracie introduced me, I recalled the trick where you calmed yourself by imagining your audience in their underwear. But the topic at hand stripped *me* bare.

I took a deep breath and plowed ahead, explaining seizures' symptoms and the differences between types of seizures I had. I stressed that I typically needed comfort and reassurance, not medical care. I answered a couple questions, and then it ended.

Sharing details about my most vulnerable self didn't cause me more embarrassment when I interacted with colleagues after that meeting. Indignation toward Tracie for imposing that task on me overpowered any shame stirred up. I saw the gesture for what it was: an unsuccessful, possibly illegal attempt to compel me to quit after I had my baby.

When I received Katherine's full-year evaluation in December, it didn't surprise me to find it both rife with negative feedback and again based on an unfair time frame. Katherine and I had formalized my new objectives two weeks earlier, but on the basis of the new objectives, her evaluation assessed my job performance for the previous twelve months.

I called the union rep Carl after work hours.

"I refuse to sign this evaluation. Katherine and I agreed to these performance objectives two weeks ago. How could I possibly meet them?"

I was livid. Carl explained I had the right to grieve the evaluation and that he would represent me at the hearing. "Okay, thanks. I want your help."

I was eight months pregnant, due in three weeks. During the days leading up to my maternity leave, I prepared for the battle I saw coming by sending myself email threads and memos I had written to Katherine and other coworkers over the preceding year.

I met with Katherine once more before my leave began. She refused to change the evaluation, and I refused to sign it. Katherine suggested colleagues noted I looked spacey during meetings and implied their perceptions interfered with my capacity to carry out my job.

Her statement left me reeling, as though I'd been knocked in the nose. It didn't match up with what I knew to be true about myself. I wanted to scream but held back.

"I always take copious notes at meetings," I pointed out again. Katherine said nothing.

The meeting was over, the negative evaluation unsigned.

When I got home, I typed up a summary of the exchange.

❧ ☙

Six days later on a gray January day, Liam was born after much coaxing. I experienced initial contractions over the previous weekend, so we went to the hospital on Sunday. They sent me home pregnant on Monday after many failed attempts at delivery.

My buddy Marilyn reminded me that acupuncture treatments can help induce labor. A professionally trained acupuncturist, she invited Mark and me to her home for treatment. I lay weary and worn on the bed she'd kindly set up, and she massaged the critical pressure points on my ankles, neck, and the webbing between my thumb and forefinger. The spots seemed unrelated to childbirth, but I eagerly wanted to try anything that might help, and the extra care felt good. I felt hopeful when we went back the hospital the next day.

My optimism waned when my labor with Liam stretched out over thirty-eight hours, an agonizing blur of pushing, pain, and exhaustion. Though I required an epidural injection of anesthetic, I avoided a C-section.

During those last excruciating minutes of labor, I gazed intently at Mark's face as I pushed from my inner core with all my might. He wore an olive-colored tee shirt, and the overhead hospital light reflected the color onto his eyes. The bright gleam turned his usually brown eyes slightly green. I focused on the color transformation and thrust as hard as I could, grunting as I did. Finally, the doctor guided Liam into this world. She handed him wailing with life up to me, and I held him to my chest as I stroked the back of his head. When he was quiet and comforted, I handed him to Mark with a triumphant smile.

I contemplated leaving MEDUSA. Liam's birth would provide a natural explanation for any resumé gap quitting might create.

I'm sure Katherine and Tracie hoped I wouldn't return when my leave ended. But Tracie's inappropriate request coupled with Katherine's lies about my performance galvanized me to stay and push back. While I didn't agree with my father's advice about hiring nannies, I sought his opinion on my job quandary. Based on his advice, I planned to return to MEDUSA, and grieve the poor evaluation. Though nationally acclaimed in their field, MEDUSA's noble mission and altruistic public face didn't jibe with its unfair management practices, which violated the Americans with Disabilities Act, ADA.

If Tracie and Katherine thought I would go down without a fight, they were sorely mistaken. In addition to my fortitude, I had my writing. My pages of careful notes and memos empowered me.

I managed initial formal grievance steps while nursing Liam and adjusting to motherhood. I had multiple email exchanges and phone meetings with my union rep Carl, Belinda from human resources, and MEDUSA's HR director, Flora. Following those emails, Carl submitted my grievance request, the unsigned evaluation, and the boatload of memos I'd sent to Katherine and human resources during the twenty months leading up to my leave.

Human resources agreed to put my grievance procedure on hold until my maternity leave ended in May. I raised the ADA discrimination issue with Carl and the other union steward, Maryanne. Though sympathetic, they said my case wasn't strong enough after checking with the union's attorney. They could assist only with grieving the unfair evaluation.

The ADA defines disability as *a physical or mental impairment that substantially limits one or more major life activities*. Passed in 1990, the law contains strong language defending disabled people's civil liberties and requiring reasonable accommodations from their employers. Before hitting that brick wall at MEDUSA, I'd only ever thought of myself as a person who had a seizure disorder. I'd thought of my epilepsy as merely a nuisance —it didn't feel disabling until MEDUSA management started hassling me about it. But in the face of MEDUSA's harassment, I was ready to wield the ADA's protective shield despite the union reps' and attorney's opinions.

I planned to grieve the evaluation *and* press the ADA issue.

I appreciated the union's support on the grievance even though I also felt like their dumped castoff: I had to manage the ADA issue solo. But I recognized MEDUSA's treatment of me since the grand mal seizure as flat out wrong. With or without the union's assistance I could call MEDUSA's illegal actions out for what they were.

Screw you all. I'm pushing this.

I went back to work in mid May and resumed the grievance procedure, a series of meetings. Carl and I met with Katherine within the week and discussed her issues with my job performance. Referencing my pages of notes, email threads, and Katherine's lack of management support, I refuted points she'd raised in her evaluation., I reminded everybody Katherine had yet to clarify which skills and knowledge I didn't have to handle the corporate outreach component.

I suspected Tracie and Katherine imagined me having a seizure while meeting with a potential corporate donor and recoiled at that image. I suggested to Carl that HR should reasonably accommodate my epilepsy by finding a different writing position that required less time interacting with outside stakeholders.

It didn't surprise me when Katherine emailed her denial a week later. I received the letter the Friday before Memorial Day weekend, and I met with Carl and the HR rep Belinda the same day.

"We're not discussing any issues related to your epilepsy—just the concerns listed in the grievance," she explained.

Shackled by Belinda's directive, I participated in the meeting focused on the same trite details: Katherine's slow responses, lack of support, and inaccurate time frames.

Over the long weekend, I sent Carl a request:

> Since the grievance procedure won't address MEDUSA's concerns about my epilepsy, MEDUSA should find another way to deal with them. Belinda and her manager can have a candid confidential discussion with me about my epilepsy and its implications regarding my managers' perceptions of my job performance.

Carl submitted my request as well as my appeal of the denial.

And then, even though Belinda had said HR wouldn't talk about the epilepsy issue—or more likely because of it—HR came forth with a deal. That week Belinda's boss Flora called me at work.

My heart rate increased when Flora announced herself on the phone. "After discussing the matter, we think a formal separation agreement would be in everybody's best interest," she said. "We're drafting something now, which I'll send you later today."

Since HR hadn't suggested an alternate MEDUSA job position, I'd come to hope for a separation agreement. I was too nervous to ask Flora about the agreement's terms while on the phone. I found out when it arrived two days later.

The draft agreement offered me five months' severance pay. In exchange, I would keep quiet about everything leading up to the settlement.

The proposed arrangement uplifted me. Despite what the union stewards had said about a discrimination lawsuit being a long shot, MEDUSA's offer signified that they took the possibility seriously. MEDUSA's proposition also infuriated me. For two years, I'd put up with a negative workplace environment and unsupportive management. My career had stagnated due to Katherine's lack of support.

I scheduled a final meeting with HR for the next day.

Carl and I met with Belinda and Flora in one of MEDUSA's sterile conference rooms. I'd attended dozens of development department meetings there over the years, but with the HR staff across the table, the fluorescently lit space felt formal and unfamiliar. Although grateful with Carl seated next to me, I was also alone. Discrimination claims weren't the union's responsibility—I had them to bear alone.

I longed for more solid support. I dreaded vetting over the same wretched details and having my professional reputation further examined under Flora and Belinda's microscope.

I kept myself from squirming by recalling my father's emailed advice: *Be strong and positive about yourself*, he'd written. I remembered the day he taught me to ride a two-wheeler. I was almost eight, and he had removed the trainers from the bicycle. He ran next to me, keeping his hand on my back as I pedaled with all my might, and I was fine until the moment I felt him take his hand away. Then I panicked and lost my balance. After countless versions of that skid-and-fall routine, I *finally* got on the bicycle feeling confident.

"Okay, one more time," Dad said, running by my side. "You can do this," he cheered, picking up on my confidence. He took his hand away, and I rode to the end of the path solo.

I looked Flora and Belinda squarely in the eye and plowed into my litany of why I couldn't accept their proposed five months' severance package.

"Stress brings on seizures, and for two years, I've put up with the constant worry that my managers were judging me because I had epilepsy. This likely increased the number of seizures I had. My career has languished during my time at MEDUSA while Katherine refused to support me on the corporate outreach project.

"MEDUSA has offered me fewer travel options due to my epilepsy. Dealing with these grievance proceedings during late pregnancy and while on maternity leave has been awful. I also don't know what's coming next professionally—my family was counting on that income.

"When you consider all this, five months' severance is insufficient," I wrapped up. "I think I deserve three years' pay." I could feel my gut wrenching slightly from nerves and anger. *Was that a slight catch I heard in my voice? Or did I imagine it?*

"It's true that Katherine has talked to us about safety concerns when you travel, due to your health condition. We agreed she should limit the number of times she asked you to take business trips," Belinda noted.

"What if we offered you a year's pay and health benefits?" Flora proposed.

I considered the proposition before me. I was offended that other than travel restraints, they hadn't addressed any of the issues I'd raised. The limited travel was the least of MEDUSA's transgressions. But in that moment, I just wanted to get out of that cold room and away from MEDUSA's probing. Despite everything left unsaid, I accepted the offer, more than double their original one.

By day's end, Flora emailed me an updated version of the separation agreement that reflected the increased severance package, which I signed and sent back.

It felt bittersweet to finalize the contract. My fight had ended. I had won, yet I felt dejected. I'd given MEDUSA my best for five years, but in the face of my epilepsy, that wasn't enough. I could handle my seizures—why the frig couldn't they?

I was exasperated.

The contract gave each party a week for recission, time to renege. After seven days with no such action, the contract went into effect. MEDUSA paid me a year's salary and benefits, and I kept quiet about their transgressions.

Despite the contract's clauses protecting me from defamation, I worried that Katherine or other MEDUSA staff might give me a bad professional reference. Although that didn't happen, I carried the stress of MEDUSA-related anxiety for years.

During that first week of summer, I received the strangest phone call. My cellphone showed a call coming from Fiona's home line. I assumed she was calling to bid me farewell after my abrupt departure. But when I answered, there was a man on the other side, explaining he was following up on a message I'd left at Disability Law Center in Boston. I'd called DLC during my ordeal and left a voicemail but stopped pursuing them after receiving other legal advice. I explained I no longer needed DLC's support, and I got off the phone as quickly as I could.

Why would somebody at DLC be calling from Fiona's home line after business hours? It didn't make any sense. Given the timing of the call, so close to when I signed the agreement with MEDUSA, I concluded MEDUSA staff asked Fiona to call me to see if I'd share any information about what had transpired. Had MEDUSA learned that I said something to the person on the line, they could have contended I'd violated the agreement. I felt paranoid. *Would Fiona set me up like that?* She had come to visit me in the hospital, after all. We were teammates for years, but I second-guessed myself for months.

Fiona and I live in adjoining neighborhoods, use the same subway stops, and frequent the same stores. Inevitably every year or two, I ran into her at a shop or on the train. We have multiple commonalities: we followed similar professional trajectories, and we are both Jewish older mothers with curly hair. Given our shared experiences, it should be effortless to start conversations when we see each other by chance. But whenever it happens, I remember that call from her landline, and I have nothing to say. *I can't believe you tried to throw me under the bus like that,* I silently scream while glaring at her.

We've had that serendipitous silent exchange multiple times since I left MEDUSA, Fiona turning her glance every time like a scared bunny. Her refusal to meet my gaze reinforces my version of what happened.

Enough time has passed that I can think about forgiving Fiona for possibly tossing me to the wolves. Toward that end, I expanded my version of Fiona's narrative a little. Perhaps she handed the phone to a friend or partner and asked him to masquerade as someone calling me from Disability Law Center. Had I shared any information with him, Fiona could honestly have said that I hadn't told her anything when asked by MEDUSA staff. Perhaps she always planned to save my butt. When I tell myself that version, I can imagine cracking a smile at her the next time I see her on the subway platform.

Child Care Calculations

I was forty when Liam was born, and despite his onerous delivery, I had an uncomplicated pregnancy. My age pushed the envelope, but I really wanted a second child in part because of my closeness as a young girl to my sister Greta. I wanted that original bestie for Liam, too—somebody with whom he could play games, create imaginary worlds, and later recall shared memories. I also wanted Liam to have a sibling at the other end, a loving comrade to assist when the time came to deal with whatever health issues Mark and I might later have. I especially wanted my kids to have each other when we passed on, as they'll likely be relatively young.

Mark was on board with the plan for two kids, so soon after Liam's birth, I started watching my cycle and marking the calendar. My plan was dicey, but Liam's pregnancy had gone well, and I was hopeful. As a grant writer, I must meet deadlines and turn in reports and requests by a specific date. As weeks ticked by, fears of age-related birth complications haunted me, so I applied professional protocols to the pregnancy: If I couldn't get pregnant in time to give birth by my forty-third birthday, I'd stop trying. Amelia arrived on May 12, 2009, exactly seven months before my deadline.

While my second pregnancy posed no more gestational complications than the first, Amelia's birth was drastically different. Where Liam needed days of coaxing and multiple attempts to lure him into this world, we feared Amelia would pop out in the car during the short drive to the hospital. Happily, we made it to Mount Auburn Hospital in Cambridge ahead of her, and Amelia was born within an hour. Triumph coursed through me as if I'd hiked Mount Everest and crested the top, from where I viewed beautiful snow-covered summits. In my hospital bed. I joyfully looked down at my healthy, beautiful daughter suckling with joy at my chest. With Mark, I had created the family I'd envisioned.

It's well-known that second labors are easier. Doctors typically attribute the phenomenon to the mother's muscle memory and increased stretching capacity after the first birth. Comparing Liam's and Amelia's labors, I also factored in my epilepsy. During my pregnancy with Amelia, I had only complex partial seizures, but I had a grand mal seizure when five months into Liam's pregnancy. Mark and I were at the health club, with the seizure big enough for Mark to take me to an ER. When I came out of it, I had nothing much to do but wait for the effects of the seizure and anticonvulsants to wear off.

Within a day, I contacted my neurologist. She increased both my medications. I didn't fall or harm myself during the seizure, and as far as I could tell, it had not affected my pregnancy in any way. But given my grueling thirty-eight-hour labor with Liam, I wonder if the in utero impact of the grand mal led to resistance on his birth day. My theory is pure speculation. I've spoken with several practitioners—mine and Liam's—over the years, and again, and with the inherent mystery of neurological disorders, nobody can say for certain.

Anybody with kids can tell you parenting truly alters your lens on the world in every way. From juggling mundane logistics of kids' extracurriculars to the impact of vacationing in one hotel room with children in the next bed, they have a pervasive effect on parents' lives. I had the added challenge of figuring out how I would parent while managing my epilepsy, but I was ready to take all of it on.

When I became a parent, I had an average of six partial complex seizures a month. We stuck with the plan I'd laid out to my neurologist and didn't hire a nanny to stay with me while Mark was at work. If on my own with the kids when I felt a seizure coming on, I generally had enough wits and time to take basic precautionary measures to safeguard them. If we walked outside, I stopped on the sidewalk and put the brakes on the stroller. Although I couldn't remember what happened during a seizure, I had enough awareness and body control that I didn't fall. I might briefly stagger in a confused circle or take a wrong turn, but I didn't trip or collide with someone or something.

My mathematical calculations about having seizures while alone with the kids proved correct, typically happening twice a month with others occurring at other times. But those equations didn't factor in my draining sense of failure each time. I lost awareness during a seizure, so obviously I wasn't doing a good job parenting in those moments. During post-seizure hazy moments, I could account for my kids' whereabouts and well-being, but I ran on autopilot and foggy for a few minutes. Sometimes I'd call Mark to ground myself in the day's routine. By the time I got on the phone, I had mostly recovered but felt weighed down by incompetence and embarrassment.

I had an innate sense about the flawed, sometimes precarious nature of caretaking in that reflexive mode. Fortunately, it never lasted long, and I always pulled through. When I came out of the foggy grasp of a seizure, I masked my deep feelings of ineptitude and guilt by focusing on whatever I was doing prior to the seizure. But I couldn't totally shake off the feelings. I comforted myself with the fact that the other ninety-nine percent of the time, I did fine.

My calculations also didn't account for other people's reactions to my seizures. As a safety precaution, I wore a medical identification bracelet that listed my condition and contact information for Mark and my neurologist. I also had a tag on the kids' stroller: *My mother has epilepsy. If you find this carriage and it appears to be abandoned, she probably had a small seizure and is in the vicinity. She will recover within a few minutes. Please call one of these numbers ASAP.* The tag listed Mark's phone numbers.

Before I was a parent, there was only one time I had a complex partial seizure in public, and an alarmed passerby called 911. Typically, my seizures ended before an observer felt compelled to call medics. My children changed that equation. Passersby sought assistance. They saw young children in my charge and me temporarily incapacitated, and they called 911. Nobody ever followed instructions on my tag and reached out to Mark.

Calling authorities was an understandable response, although I hated dealing with the aftermath. The situation arose about ten times when the kids were young. One summer day, I took Liam downtown on the subway. He was still an infant, harnessed against my chest in a baby carrier, and I was grateful for his body heat on the overly air-conditioned train.

As we rode home from Boston, brain turmoil took over beyond Kendall Square, Cambridge. It started out as a creeping sensation in my tummy that edged upward. Eventually, my face tingled, too, and I knew the seizure wouldn't stop. The last thing I remember was the relief I felt as I noted the relatively empty subway car—at least not many people would witness what would come next.

I imagine my fellow passengers saw this: a confused woman with a baby. Possibly she smacked her lips and moaned out loud. When the train arrived at Central Square, she exited the subway and she pushed her stroller, her baby strapped to her chest. In the throes of the seizure, I followed my primal embarrassed instincts and dashed off the train. I was still spacey, but I desperately wanted to get away from my fellow riders. Although staying on the subway would have been the safest thing to do, I couldn't bear to be near the other passengers while knowing they witnessed me in such an exposed and vulnerable state.

I sat on a bench at the Central Square underground platform, Liam on my chest, his stroller next to me as we waited for the next train. My stomach relaxed a bit as my body normalized. I checked my watch repeatedly, something I frequently did post seizure to ground myself. When an EMT approached me on the platform, I determined that somebody on the train must have called 911.

"Are you okay?" he asked.

"Yes, I am now." I explained what had happened, then completed required forms verifying that I didn't need medical attention. The medic left the station, and I waited with Liam for the next northbound train toward home. Although I understood why he was called in, managing the medic's intervention added weight on top of Liam's body on my front and the baby bag slung on my back, as I recovered from the seizure I just had.

Minutes later, the train arrived and I boarded the subway car far away from people waiting near me. Nobody in my car had a clue about what had just happened. To them, I was just a middle-aged, curly-haired mother out on a jaunt with her cute baby. By the end of the eight-minute ride, the post-seizure fog had totally lifted. I walked back home from Davis Square and put Liam to sleep for his nap.

With passersby scared enough to call medics, I questioned whether the risk I took was too big. Clearly, I appeared off balance enough to others that people felt concerned for Liam's and my safety that day. A gushing waterfall of guilt poured over me as I thought about what *may* have happened. An ill-intentioned passerby *could* have done something evil to both of us. I looked at Liam sleeping in his crib and took in his tranquil form and steady breathing. I squeezed his tiny foot and relished the feel of his delicate toes. Nothing nefarious had happened—the proof was in the crib.

At dinner, I relayed the story to Mark with Liam strapped in his highchair, slamming his hand on the table, and interspersing our conversations with gleeful yelping.

"I was fine by the time the medics got to the Central Square platform. Well, aware anyway. I was embarrassed and a little shaken, and Liam was squirming in his papoose, but I was ready to go home."

"Did the medics offer to take you?"

"No. Once I signed paperwork verifying that I was okay, they left, which was fine. We took the next subway."

"And no more seizures after that?"

"No. I've been fine. It's just upsetting to think about what bad things *could* happen when I'm out of it. I feel like a bad mother."

"You're not. Nothing bad happened—remember that. It's not helpful to dwell on the negative might-haves," Mark said.

Mark was correct that nothing bad happened that day nor ever before or after when I had seizures while out with my children. Years later, Mark told me he harbored some concerns about the kids' safety—a bit of worry that nagged at him in the background. But during the kids' early years, his optimistic outlook was critical to getting our family through the challenges. And while dealing with medics primarily stoked embarrassment, resentment, and resignation, gratitude mixed in. I knew those 911 calls were a safety measure and a sign of strangers' kindness, and I appreciated both.

Walking toward Davis Square a few years later, I pushed our red double stroller with three-year-old Liam on top and Amelia—less than a year old at that time—tucked in the seat beneath him. As we neared the pasta shop, telltale flutters stirred in my stomach followed by dreaded creeping sensations across my mouth and face.

I put the brake on the stroller and leaned against the nearby storefront. *Just breathe*, I instructed myself, attempting to stave off my anxiety. Sometimes internal coaching warded off the grip of a complex partial seizure. On those lucky days, deep breathing kept me grounded, and I experienced only minor seizure symptoms: tummy flutters, creeping sensations, and watch-checking during episodes known as simple seizures.

That day wasn't a lucky one. Brain chaos got the better of me as sensations across my face progressed to something bigger. I lost awareness and fell off the complex partial seizure cliff, so I don't know what others saw. Maybe mouth smacking, maybe erratic pacing or shaking—something odd enough to trigger a bystander's alarm. When the seizure subsided and I regained awareness, an ambulance's flashing lights distracted me. As medics questioned me I felt slightly woozy and rattled to my core by the seizure. I signed the paperwork and assured them I didn't need medical care.

By wild coincidence, my brother Daniel had run a work-related errand at Dave's Pasta and was right in front of the shop as the medics left. Daniel walked us to the post office and chatted about our relatives as we strolled through the square.

Daniel lived only about twenty-five miles from me, but despite our proximity, we weren't that close. I hadn't seen him in a few months. While it was a bummer that our chance visit took place under such nerve-wracking circumstances, I was relieved that Daniel didn't make a huge deal about them. By nature, he was not an emotional gusher and sometimes seemed distant, and that day I felt grateful for his discretion.

I purchased my stamps, and Daniel walked me out of the post office.

"You okay?" he asked.

"Yeah, I'm fine. I've got to get Amelia home for her nap." They were both true statements. Daniel took them at face value and gave me a parting hug. I took the kids home.

The drive to continue comprised a critical piece of my normalizing post-seizure strategy. The more efficiently I assimilated, I figured, the less impact the seizure had on my morale. Misfiring neurons may have gotten the better of my brain and subsequently slammed me with a one-two punch, but like a champion boxer, I came back—a little spacey, perhaps in need of extra coffee, but ready to go. At least that's what I told myself, and that's how I buoyed my self esteem.

While I didn't need medical care after a complex partial seizure, the best recovery measures would have included an extended restful break—say twenty minutes on a soft couch or sunny park bench. But taking additional time would have meant appearing abnormal for that much longer. My choice to operate on autopilot during post-seizure haze was a subconscious intuitive instinct—a defense mechanism to sidestep shameful feelings when others had witnessed my temporary incapacitation. Avoiding embarrassment at all costs was paramount, even if it meant increased safety risks.

My kids were likely too young to remember those specific days, but they witnessed dozens of my seizures over time. For them, living with an awareness that something could go wrong with Mom seemed as big a challenge as observing the seizures. The children became hyper-sensitive to my first outward seizure symptoms, often an involuntary scared moan combined with a sharp intake of breath.

One evening, we were all on the couch in the living room reading stories before bed. I'd had a long day, and I was tired. I inhaled sharply, emitting an audible sigh as I let my breath go. Then I saw Liam's automatic response kick in as his body tensed and he anxiously glanced my way.

"I'm okay—I'm not having a seizure," I reassured him, eager to assuage his worry. He refocused on Mark's voice reading Dr. Seuss's soothing rhythms.

Rather than assuaging my concerns, their increased independence shifted them as the children matured. I felt less apprehensive about physical harm such as accidental falls and more uneasy about the emotional impact that witnessing my seizures might have on them. When they were old enough to put words to the situation, we talked about what had happened.

"You had a seizure," Liam observed after the fact as I resurfaced from the grip of a complex partial seizure. He was about six at the time.

"Yes, I did. I'm okay now," I reassured him. "Are you two okay?" I asked. I wanted to give them the opportunity to vent about their fears, although they rarely did.

"We're fine," Liam said.

"You went the wrong way on the street," Amelia observed. We had been walking home from school on quiet side streets when the seizure started. In my confusion, I hung a right toward the cul-de-sac instead of heading left toward home. When I resurfaced, I had reoriented as we continued the short walk toward the house.

"Yeah, we took the long way home, didn't we? Sorry about that."

The kids didn't know it, but I apologized for far more than the small detour. I was sorry that once again they had to witness me lost in my internal chaotic seizure state without another grownup around to assure them everything would be okay. Watching it surely frightened them. Guilt washed over me and left me subdued. Once home, I distracted the kids with television and myself with dinner prep. I finely chopped vegetables for a big batch of tomato sauce, the knife's blade rhythmically slamming against the cutting board as I minced onions, garlic, mushrooms, and peppers. Unlike my neurological wiring, vegetable chopping offered something I could control. I immersed myself in the task.

Although I hadn't physically left their sides, I'd briefly abandoned Liam and Amelia on the way home just as I had every time I'd had a seizure while alone with them. Like a brick sailing through a glass window shattering it to shards, the reality bashed my good-mom self-image. I focused on the tomato sauce, which smelled delicious. Dinner was going to be great.

As I'd predicted, having seizures while alone with the kids wasn't easy or good for any of us, but it was tolerable—risky, of course, but infrequent enough that although I was concerned and cautious, I wasn't alarmed. Based on my own life experience, I found parenting manageable while coping with my seizures. By default, my kids acquired enough courage to witness their mother's seizures—surely an unfair imposition but with a certain up side. For the kids, I imagine my aimless walk home that day felt like drifting over rocky waters atop a rickety raft. As the grip of the seizure loosened and my equilibrium returned, they saw the raft still floating, and they could relax.

Over the years, I've apologized multiple times for forcing them to put up with my epilepsy. I hugged them tightly as I explained that my only other option was not to have them, and I couldn't bear that. When she was eleven, Amelia and I had an iteration of the discussion where she bluntly called out my choice.

"You knew you would have seizures when you borned me. That was a selfish thing to do." Amelia's ungrammatical form of "birth" moved me. "Borned" was a word she'd coined years earlier, and we'd incorporated it into our family lexicon. Her correct accusation stirred me, and I needed to validate it.

"You're right. It was. I'm sorry you had to experience so many of my scary seizures when you were young. I'm still glad I had you and Liam. Are you glad you're here?"

Amelia nodded.

"Good. Come here."

We sat side by side at the dining room table, and she popped off her chair, happy to be scooped into my arms.

I'd gotten through the other side of a childhood full of insecurities, including seizures. Amelia and Liam clearly inherited some of my resilience. For the first few years of their lives, I thought their strength combined with the support I provided the other ninety-nine percent of the time and the scaffolding Mark and I offered were enough. Such loving, careful planning and precautions would get us through tenuous scary moments brought on by my seizures.

Until the day came when I knew that wasn't true.

Fostering Resilience

Although epilepsy added challenging—sometimes alarming— aspects to parenting, I never doubted my ability to take them on. As a kid I'd assimilated to multiple insecurities, starting with my body and my family.

My mother recounted seeing me in the throes of something resembling seizure activity when I was a baby, but I wasn't officially diagnosed with epilepsy until I was six. At the time, we were living in apartment 1B of the Lefrak City apartment complex, in Queens. Sprawling across forty acres, Lefrak was comprised of forty-six hundred units. Everything residents needed was there—stores, library, school, playgrounds, even the doctor's office. My mother, baby sister, and I had moved there about a year and a half earlier after my parents' divorce.

My parents split up when I was four. My only memory of their marriage is the wretched screaming matches they had in our previous apartment on the fifteenth floor of the same building. Apartment 1B was smaller and riddled with cockroaches—we had moved down in every way. Whenever I turned on the kitchen light, bugs scuttled across the pale yellow linoleum tiles and disappeared into the crevices where the cabinet met the floor. The at-large cockroaches unnerved me almost as much as Mom's suitors.

"Get away from her, you leech!" Mom's boyfriend Roger screamed at my baby sister Greta. She wasn't even two and still drinking from bottles, clinging to our mother's side. Roger was jealous of the attention Mom paid to her. He also spanked us hard if he heard us playing games after bedtime.

There was Mr. Steckler, bald with thick black cat-eye-framed glasses. Mr. Steckler offered us nickels, pieces of bubble gum, and boxes of candied popcorn. Although I enjoyed these gifts, his manner was hushed and awkward, and I knew he was only there to see my mother. I never learned his first name.

Greta and I shared the small bedroom, and Mom slept on the living room foldout. When Mom put us to bed, images of cockroaches creeping on the sheets kept me awake. On nights Roger wasn't there, I waited for the sound of Mom opening the couch. I was eager for the comfort of her company. But I couldn't leave Greta alone—the cockroaches might crawl into her bed—so I carried her to Mom's bed. After I checked the front door to make sure all the locks were fastened, I climbed onto the foldout double bed next to Greta and Mom. Then I felt safe enough to crash into a deep slumber.

One day, I was in my bedroom playing with my two-dimensional plastic tiles, the set a present for my sixth birthday. The multi-colored plastic rectangles were smooth on one side and had short stubby pegs that fit into a light blue plastic board lined with rows of holes. I placed the tiles in a random design. As I admired the display of color, I felt the queerest sensation in my stomach.

What is that? I wondered. I felt pressure, but no nausea. It was simply weird.

I looked around my small room, taking comfort in the familiarity. Everything was where it should be: the matching twin beds with white wooden frames on opposite walls, the brightly colored toy chest with cheerful bunny decals in the corner. But something was off inside me. The pressure in my tummy ratcheted up a couple notches as if I'd been socked in the stomach. Fear raced through me. I was free falling with nobody to catch me. I was still in my room but on a gut level I had lost my grip on the world. Panicking, I looked out my bedroom door. I could see into the kitchen, where Mom was cooking. I wanted to go to her, but the short distance seemed insurmountable. "Mom!" I screamed as the grand mal seizure's impact hit me full force.

Then I blanked out.

My mother apparently called an ambulance. As my mother and father arrived, I woke up the next day in nearby Elmhurst General

Hospital. They both wore full-length black wool coats. Their coordinated outerwear spurred a fleeting optimistic thought: *Maybe their matching coats are a sign that my parents can stay together.* I recalled their raging fights and recognized my hope as pure fantasy. Reality was the cockroaches and my mother's boyfriends in our basement apartment. But it made me happy to bask in their eager concerned greetings. My mother grinned ear to ear, thrilled when she saw I was awake.

"You're up!" she exclaimed. Even my typically reserved father grabbed me in a clumsy bear hug as he approached the hospital bed.

"How you feeling?" he asked.

"Better." Compared to the previous day's physical mayhem, the ache in my head felt minor. Too young to grasp the long-term implications of an epilepsy diagnosis, I understood something was amiss with my body or I wouldn't be in the hospital— that's where sick people went when something was wrong with them.

Would I be back here again, soon? I sure hoped not.

❧ ☙

After that seizure, the doctors sent me home with a prescription for phenytoin. The yellow triangular tablets were mint-flavored like peppermint candies. I cheered myself up by pretending I was eating a sweet treat when I took the pills. But I found absolutely nothing fun about getting blood tests to check drug levels. I flinched and cried out from needle pricks—even when Mom held my hand, but her presence comforted me. She dutifully sought doctors' advice and smiled optimistically when they suggested the seizures might stop.

Time-consuming, onerous, and isolating electroencephalograms or EEGs constituted a different brand of painful. I sat in a big chair while a technician measured and marked my head with a special pen, applied glue on the red Xs drawn, and then stuck twenty electrodes to my scalp. I followed the technician's instructions—gazing at flashing strobe lights, closing my eyes while hyperventilating. For half an hour, they recorded activity of my brain waves. Then they sent me home with ink blotches on my forehead and glue caked into my thick curls, already prone to snarls. Mom and I were near tears by the time we completely removed the gooey paste and stubborn ink.

A couple months after the first seizure, I had another grand mal. I was with Dad on a weekend visit at his friends' home in suburban New Jersey.

The Victors lived in a white house with a lawn. My father brought my sister and me there most weekends in the months following the divorce. I loved the visits. I was eager to see our father, as it provided reassurance that he still loved us even though he'd moved out.

Visits to the Victors' home also provided a peek into the family life I yearned for: a light airy house with enough bedrooms for everybody and an intact family, including Susan, a mother who had the patience to comb out my curly mop and pin it up into thick Teddy bear-ear pigtails.

There were also kids to play with, as the Victor family had two sons. Adam was my age and Jonathan two years older. Adam and Jonathan seemed smart and sophisticated. I longed for their acceptance. We played competitive board and card games. I was always trying to prove myself, but it felt hopeless.

During our visits, the adults ensconced themselves upstairs in the living room. Good music, food, and dope were the orders of their day. My father was dating Mary, whom he would eventually marry, and she joined us at the Victors'.

We kids retreated to the basement rec room and debated about how to entertain ourselves.

"Let's play Flintstones. I'll be Wilma. You can be Fred," I suggested to Adam.

"Eeew no way! Let's just watch television," he said.

"There's *Sesame Street*," I suggested.

"That's for babies," Jonathan scorned. I didn't dare let on that it was still one of my favorite shows. "We like *Pink Panther* and *Superheroes*."

"*Pink Panther*'s okay. I like the *Flintstones* and *Scooby Doo*, too," I said.

"Yeah, *Scooby Doo* is cool," Adam agreed, and I basked in the scrap of positive reinforcement.

We were on the floor watching Bugs Bunny when I felt the clenching sensation in my stomach. This time I knew what it was. Initially, I focused on immediate details: the rec room's familiar wood paneling, the metal antenna poked up from behind the television like thin rabbit ears. I combed the brown shag carpet between my fingers and leaned against the low wood frame of the waterbed.

I glanced at Adam and Jonathan. They were riveted to Elmer Fudd futilely chasing Bugs. They had no idea what was happening to me.

Then the weird sensations spread across my face with a tingling on the surface of my lips. Despite my acute awareness of carpet threads and wood panels, I was losing my hold on the world.

There was no hiding it from Jonathan and Adam. Already on the floor, I couldn't fall, yet I felt the rug shifting under my legs and butt. I looked helplessly at the boys, who seemed frightened. In retrospect, I realize the boys knew the floor wasn't moving, but they probably saw some odd twitching or jerking movements in my body. In that moment, they knew something was wrong, and I was too panicked to feel embarrassed.

"Get my dad," I pleaded, grateful to see Adam already scampering up the stairs. And the grownups apparently responded, although I was oblivious by the time they came downstairs. The next thing I knew I was post-seizure and woozy at Morristown Medical Center. I would have said it felt like a rip roaring hangover, but at the time I didn't yet know that phrase. Instead, I noticed enormous pain in my forehead and an off-kilter sensation like my head was too big for the rest of my body.

My father brought me home the next day and passed on the attending doctor's instructions. "They said Laura needs an appointment with her neurologist at Mount Sinai. They probably need to change her medications."

"Okay. I'll call them tomorrow," Mom said. "How are you feeling, honey?" She extended her arm toward me as she squatted down to embrace me in a hug.

"I'm okay." Relieved to breathe in her familiar sweet scent and to see my parents interacting nicely with each other, I relaxed into my mother's hold.

We met with the doctor shortly after. He suggested adding a second medication. Eager to take any measure necessary to avert the random scary episodes, my mother readily agreed.

Other than some occasional bouts of lethargy, the medication didn't have major side effects. Best of all, the seizures stopped for a few years. I still had to take pills twice daily, make bi-annual pilgrimages to Mount Sinai in Manhattan, and undergo burdensome EEGs every year, but the seizures were under control. From the outsider's perspective, I appeared *normal*, which was a huge relief.

※ ※

The summer before my seventh birthday, we moved to the Bronx. Bolton Street was around the corner from the elevated train stop on Pelham Parkway and White Plains Road. At night we could hear the Number 5 trains rattling by at all hours, but it wasn't long before I could tune the rumbles out as background white noise. The new apartment was a definite step up. Our unit was on the fourth floor, which felt safer, as it was several stories above ground level. Boogeymen were less likely to climb through our windows, and although we still had cockroaches, they weren't nearly as prevalent.

Despite the seizure respite and upgraded living conditions, I still didn't feel *normal* during elementary school. Although I wasn't having seizures, the experience instilled a subconscious body insecurity. I didn't dwell on it, but the possibility of having a seizure lurked, and the awareness created an intuitive self-doubt.

During those years, my kinky curly hair made me feel more ostracized than the epilepsy did. Tight curls have never fit the conventional American beauty mold, and I despised my hair. All the dolls had stick straight blonde dos. The television icons —from Wonder Woman to Cher to Elizabeth Montgomery's *Bewitched* - all had neat orderly coifs. I spent countless frustrated hours blow drying it trying to get the curls to disappear, which never worked. The blow dryer and straighteners left my curls slightly more relaxed, but my hair was still bulky and frizzy. My straight-haired mother was clueless about how to style my locks, so eventually I agreed to cut it short. My do resembled a slightly browner version of Little Orphan Annie's.

On top of corkscrew curls and daily drug regimens, our family had inordinate amounts of domestic discord. I knew other kids who also had divorced parents (eventually the Victors' perfect family fell apart, too), but our family took divisiveness to a new level. The summer we moved to the Bronx, my mother married her most recent suitor, Geoffrey.

Their wedding was a large, formal affair. My mother sewed her own elegant white wedding dress and donned a diaphanous veil. She had also sewn full-length flower girl dresses for Greta and me. We looked adorable in our matching frocks—the flowing skirts decorated with turquoise, white, and green stripes, the bodices shimmery blue.

Geoffrey and my mother married in a synagogue, and I cried as they walked down the aisle. I knew that unlike her previous boyfriends, Geoffrey was here to stay. My mother's relatives thought my weeping sweet—they presumed I cried tears of joy—but I felt distraught by what I knew was coming.

Over six feet tall, Geoffrey was imposing. He wore his black hair long, often pulled back in a ponytail. Geoffrey worked at D'Agostino's grocery store. In his spare time, he smoked dope, watched television, and bought horseracing tickets at the off-track betting site around the corner. We were at odds with each other from the get-go: Geoffrey wanted to be the man of the house, and I wouldn't let him forget that I already had a father. Geoffrey issued disciplinary directives like ordering me to stop spinning on the swiveling living room chair and threatening to spank me if I didn't listen.

"You can't hit me. You're not my father," I retorted. But I got off the chair before I got whacked. It went downhill from there. My mother urged me to make more effort to get along with Geoffrey. I tried to mollify the situation by calling Geoffrey Dad for a while like Greta did. But directed at Geoffrey, the word Dad felt awkward and clunky rolling off my tongue.

For years, my biological parents put Greta and me smack in the middle of their fights over money. Their divorce agreement outlined my father's alimony and child support payments and generous visitation rights, which he was eager to leverage. After he remarried, Dad went through a back-to-the-land phase where he left his information technology career, lived in New England, and did odds-and-ends jobs to make money. During those years, he didn't rake in the dough, so sometimes he neglected to follow the divorce agreement.

One day, I heard Mom again yelling at Dad on the phone.

"You still owe me a hundred this month. I'm not going to let you take the kids for their visit until you pay it!"

Over the years, I'd heard numerous iterations of that fight.

My father shouted something in response that I couldn't make out.

"Fine!" my mother screamed back and slammed down the phone.

"Are we gonna visit with Dad this weekend?" I asked meekly.

"If he doesn't pay what he owes, he doesn't deserve to see you," my mother stormed.

My heart sank at the prospect of missing a visit. Despite Dad's gruff manner, I enjoyed our visits and wanted to see him. I didn't care about breached child support agreements. All I knew was my father hadn't entirely met his obligation, and my mother used visitation with Greta and me as collateral. I had no control over either of my parents' choices, but they could mess up my visits with Dad. Being in the middle sucked.

"I really want to go," I implored.

"Well, your father owes us money. If he pays, you can go."

Dad always showed up at the appointed visit time no matter how contentious those phone conversations. My parents then had hushed discussions, but in the end, Mom always let us go with Dad.

I was so eager for that thread of continuity with my father that I easily overlooked the hard parts of being away from home. I missed my mother when we visited for more than a weekend. Then there were the car drives. Four hours on the thruways through New York and New England seemed interminable.

"How much longer until we get there?" I'd ask an hour or so into the trip, and my father would tell me. A couple hours and several highways later, if I asked a second time, my father would grouse, "Don't be a nudge."

I entertained myself while Greta slept. Hours later, we arrived travel-weary and hungry at Dad's,. Dad had married Mary, and they had a son, Daniel. I was only vaguely interested in my new baby brother—I did not find infants interactive enough.

Mary was as warm and fuzzy as a porcupine —she had Daniel calling her by her first name by the time he was four. Her analytical cool nature was on the opposite side of the emotional spectrum from my mother's overreactive demeanor. Looking back, I think Dad chose Mary because she was everything my mother was not: detached and commonsensical to the point of dispassionate.

The cuisine at Dad's also left me longing for home. The original *Vegetarian Epicure* and *Moosewood* cookbooks were the rage, and our father was gung-ho about eating all whole grain and sugar free. His bulgur and black beans with molasses was a far cry from Mom's sloppy Joes with instant white rice.

After a meal, I longed to turn on some cartoons, but Dad and Mary had permanently stored their television in the attic— they thought it would inhibit Daniel's development. During long afternoons, I yearned for the upbeat Flintstones' opening ditty. Instead, NPR's *All Things Considered* melancholy theme resounded from the kitchen.

Various adaptions—to my body, my parents' divorce and subsequent remarriages, homes away from home, my curls — shaped my core. I was resilient, and in the face of my seizures, I was brave by default. I brought the traits to parenting, and—for better and for worse—forced them onto our children.

Adam and Jonathan were about seven and nine years old the day I had the grand mal in their rec room. Although the boys were a good deal older than my children during most of the seizures they'd witnessed, I remember the fear in Adam and Jonathan's faces that day. The seizures Amelia and Liam observed weren't nearly as severe. Our situation was challenging—sometimes scary, even- but during their early childhood years, I felt confident we could get through the nuisance and disruption my seizures brought on.

Until I was blindsided by another uptick in my brain's chaos.

The Tipping Point

The children weren't with me the day I determined seizures and parenting were an untenable combination. Liam and Amelia were four and six years old at the time and attending a summer day camp. My friend Joyce picked them up for me, so I had time to run errands at the end of my work day. I emerged from the air-conditioned store, and by the time I walked a mere block, my thighs were coated in sweat despite the breeze blowing around my flowy short skirt.

Then I felt the telltale tingling sensations in my belly kick in. Joyce didn't expect me for an hour. I had time to heed the warning of those disconcerting tummy flutters. *Okay, find a safe place to wait the seizure out.* I took refuge on the steel bench in Davis Square Plaza and focused on the granite statues nearby. There were sculptures of an elderly man and woman, their arms linked affectionately. I tried to take comfort in familiarity. It was my neighborhood. The omnipresent statues' bronzed faces kindly watched over the square —and me.

As I rested under the statues' benevolent gazes, I was unaware that the misfiring neurons in my head covered a bigger than usual section of my brain. Suddenly I was hurled into the depths of a grand mal seizure, grasped by its internal seismic shifts, completely unaware of my surroundings.

I have no memory of the time following my descent off that cliff. Based on what my family and friends have told me over the years, I imagine it looked *something* like this: during the seizure's initial moments, I wandered in an aimless circle around the plaza, an irrepressible moan forced out of my spasming body, my tongue clicking, my body shaking uncontrollably before collapsing on the sidewalk. Perhaps my limbs jerked wildly of their own accord. No doubt I was a scary sight to behold.

Typically, the greater the neurological brain chaos, the bigger the seizure is, the more perceptible the symptoms are to an onlooker. Not surprisingly, somebody in the square called 911. I was unconscious when the medics arrived, placed me on a gurney, and took me by ambulance to the local hospital.

Davis Square Plaza is smack in the middle of a six-street intersection I know well. When I came to, I could visualize the multiple traffic bottlenecks that built up on the streets when the ambulance pulled up next to the plaza and turned on its hazard lights. I could envision long lines of cars streaming on College Avenue, Holland Street, Highland Avenue, and Day Street while medics transferred me into the vehicle. I could imagine the ambulance subsequently speeding down Elm Street, lights flashing and siren blaring.

I deduced all that when a couple hours later I resurfaced from the grip of the seizure and found myself in the emergency room of Somerville Hospital. Dizzy from the effects of the anticonvulsant cocktail the doctors administered, I recovered in the hospital bed. I had a colossal headache, but I called Joyce who had already figured out what had happened. She knew I wouldn't run that late without calling without an emergency, and in that event, she knew the high probability of a seizure.

I called Mark at work. Although I had adjusted to the pain in my head, I couldn't shake the dread over my circumstance.

"I had a grand mal seizure on my way home," I said nervously. "Somebody called 911, and I'm at Somerville Hospital."

"Where are Liam and Amelia?"

"With Joyce. She picked them up from camp today—I was on my way to her house when the seizure started."

"Are you okay?".

"Kind of. I mean, my head is spinning, and I don't know why I had a grand mal, so I'm scared. But I'm not injured. Just a scratched knee. I want to go home now."

"Okay, I'll leave work as soon as I can, get the car, and meet you at the hospital. Hang tight."

When the hospital discharged me with a three-page handout about seizures, their causes, effects, and how to treat them, I accepted the impersonal offering and tried to disguise my disdain. There was nothing on that fact sheet that I didn't already know—I could have written it myself.

By the time we got home and Mark retrieved the kids from Joyce, I still felt woozy, so I retreated to my room while he fed them dinner. As I rested in bed, the enormity of the afternoon's episode sank in. Like the grand mal I had eight years before at my office, the afternoon's seizure blindsided me. It was the first one I'd had in years and for no obvious reason, a fact that nagged at me. Initially a distant pesky feeling, the troublesome awareness overshadowed the physical pain in my head. *What if the kids had been with me this afternoon?*

I recalled that, when Liam was born, I'd attached a tag to our stroller explaining that I had epilepsy and that if the carriage appeared abandoned, it was because I'd likely had a small seizure. The tag said I would "recover within a few minutes." That afternoon, the statement would have been flat out wrong.

When I replayed the scene with the kids added to the scenario, it wasn't logistics or even safety concerns that haunted me. Had Amelia and Liam been with me, I'm confident that Davis Square passersby would have figured out a way to ensure the kids' safety until family, friends, or authorities arrived.

What plagued me for weeks was imagining Liam and Amelia witnessing my uncontrolled state and calling out in fear while the grip of a grand mal incapacitated me. I could not have responded to their cries for comfort. The vision opposed my self image of good parent that I took pride in. I was asking too much of them.

Thankful that others cared for my children on that sultry July day, I knew it was pure luck that protected them from witnessing their mother completely knocked out by the one-two punch. Had they been with me, they may have been held temporarily in police custody. The image of Liam and Amelia whisked away in a patrol car to the West Somerville precinct station while I was out cold gave me shivers.

I could no longer rely on fate. It was time to consider my neurologist's recommendation for brain surgery. During our next appointment, I stepped beyond my fears and made an appointment for week-long, twenty-four-hour intensive brain-wave monitoring, the first of many tests that would lead me to a neurosurgeon's table multiple times.

Taking the Plunge

Different neurologists suggested brain surgery to me multiple times as far back as 1992. Twenty-one years and three neurologists later, I had no choice but to accept the drastic option as a possible solution. The thought of doctors cutting my head open still terrified me, but I couldn't afford to have grand mal seizures while alone with the kids. About a month after I landed in the Somerville Hospital ER. my neurologist Dr. P arranged for the first step, a long-term monitoring EEG.

She scheduled it for Monday, August 19, and I received an eight-page explanation packet. I was to stay inpatient at Brigham and Women's for from three to seven days. They'd hook me up to an EEG monitor that recorded my brain waves in front of a camera that taped my every move. The procedure would capture real-time seizure activity on video and EEG.

The doctors would try to induce a seizure by withholding my medication at some point during the stay, a tactic that concerned me. In addition to bringing on seizure activity within twenty-four hours, skipping medication also often triggered seizures from ten to twenty days later. I sent Dr. P an email.

> In an effort to avoid decreasing the meds . . . I wonder if I can take seizure-inducing measures during (or even the day before) my hospital stay. Perhaps I can make sure I get a crummy night's sleep on August 18. Or I can skip a meal or two while I'm there, to lower my blood sugar. Or focus on as many stressful things as possible—kind of a counter meditation measure.

Any of my suggested tactics would have fewer longer-term impacts than tinkering with the medication levels. Dr. P thought those measures worth trying but reiterated that if I didn't have a seizure within the first couple days, they'd resort to withholding medication.

On August 19 Mark accompanied me to the hospital for the check-in but went to work on a regular schedule for the week. My father and Chris agreed to take the kids for the week in Portland, Maine.

Hospital personnel escorted me to the fifth floor of Brigham, where the technician used old-fashioned EEG leads which she pasted to my head with gooey gel. Electrodes in place, I was led to a private room on the tenth floor and hooked up to video surveillance equipment. The camera had a cord long enough that I could go to the bathroom in private, but that was all. No showers allowed with electrodes. They instructed me to press a button if I felt anything resembling seizure activity.

Then the waiting began.

By the end of the second day, I'd had two complex partial seizures, both beginning with typical clenching in my belly. I obediently pressed the call button. When I came out of the seizures, I felt a perverse delight in addition to my typical post-seizure haze. As required, the team had recorded the seizures. But Dr. P wanted to capture a third one on tape, so on Thursday morning, they withheld my meds. I checked my emails and thought about stressful things. I'd lined up a new consulting job for September. *What if I can't find childcare in time? What if I have a backfire seizure during my first few days on the job thanks to this medication withholding?*

The third seizure started on Friday afternoon as they removed the electrodes. *At least they got it on video,* but the timing exasperated me. The doctor gave me extra levetiracetam, and I thought they might keep me overnight. During the intake, they had said something about a twelve-hour seizure-free requisite before sending patients home, but I went home woozy the same day.

In September, I learned from Dr. P that the monitoring revealed abnormalities in the right temporal lobe indicated by rhythmic slowing and spike-wave activity during seventy percent of the time the EEG tracked me. Given that number and my recent seizure patterns, it was likely only a matter of time before I had a grand mal while alone with the kids.

Dr. P was visibly pleased when I accepted her recommendation to meet with the neurosurgeon.

I was launched into the next phase of the brain surgery trajectory.

Later that month, Dr. P joined me at the preliminary meeting with Dr. A We discussed pros and cons of laser surgery versus open surgery. Though less invasive, laser surgery had lower efficacy rates, so I ruled it out. If I were going to do it, I wanted the highest success rate possible. Dr. A repeated the success rate statistic of seventy percent, with additional people whose seizure rates improved though they still had them.

"So, thirty percent of people still have them?" I asked.

"Yes. But remember, there are other risks besides seizures if you don't have the surgery."

"Like what?"

"Tests show that your seizures are focalized almost entirely on the right side of your brain. If you don't have the surgery, that focal point could shift to the left side."

"So, you're saying the bad side could corrupt the good side?"

"Something like that. The more seizures you have involving the right temporal lobe, the more likely it is that the left side of your brain will learn that activity. Also, the severity of your seizures may increase."

"What about memory loss or personality change caused by the brain surgery?" I asked.

"Personality change is uncommon, but memory loss can be an issue. Your medical history indicates that your seizures' focal point is not near the part of your brain responsible for memory. We will run tests to confirm that prior to scheduling the surgery."

"Okay, I need to think about it some more." Although Dr. A's counsel left me vaguely reassured, she could say nothing to dispel my grief. I was heartbroken that the best solution for stopping my seizures involved something so severe—the equivalent of brain dismemberment. Dr. A had a very logical calm demeanor—good for a brain surgeon, a friend later reminded me—but ineffectual for comforting the ache in my heart.

Sitting across from Dr. A, I didn't mention the pit of angst in my belly.

❧ ☙

I avoided distress and self pity by immersing myself in research into brain surgery. Over the next five months, I met with three different practitioners. I thought it worth the sixty-mile pilgrimage to Providence, Rhode Island, for consultation with Dr. R, considered the pioneer of temporal lobectomy, the operation Dr. A suggested. Despite all the advice I'd received from the Brigham and Women's team, I was scared—I needed additional confirmation. If Dr. R recommended surgery, I would probably go through with it. Since he had devised the operation, maybe he might perform it instead of Dr. A, I mused. Then I imagined scalpels near my head as I lay on a surgeon's table and felt sick with fear. What if surgery didn't work? What if I came out worse for it? No matter how experienced Dr. R, he couldn't give me the success guarantee I wanted.

The Providence trip launched my information scavenger hunt. I brought a voice recorder, a notebook, and the dark green spiral bound notebook I stored beneath my nightstand. The journal's cover was tattered with age, its wire spine reinforced with packing tape. It contained my chicken scratch records of every seizure I'd had since 2001 and notes from all my doctors' appointments over the years.

With his prominent nose, trim mustache, and receding hairline, Dr. R looked like an aging Sonny Bono. I gave him the nutshell summary of my case: refractory complex partial seizures since I was six even after trying seventeen different medications and multiple alternative therapies.

Mark and I sat on the other side of his desk in his fluorescently lit office as I rattled off all my fears and what-ifs about memory loss, failed procedures, and personality changes. Although simply reiterating what all the others had told me, I found Dr. R's avuncular manner comforting.

No, there was no guarantee brain surgery would stop the seizures. But if my most recent magnetic resonance imaging, MRI, scan confirmed that the abnormalities in my brain concentrated on one side, he would highly recommend having a right temporal

71

lobectomy. I had Dr. P's office send my MRI results to Dr. R, and after reviewing them, he too concluded that I was an "excellent" candidate for brain surgery.

The onus was then on me to decide.

I mulled for two weeks. I listened multiple times to Dr. R's voice on the appointment's taped recording as he addressed my fears: the doctors would perform a multitude of pre-tests, enabling them to pinpoint exactly which part of my brain to remove and confirm that I'd be unlikely to lose memory.

Dr. R cited the same seventy percent success rate as Dr. P and said chances were eighty-five percent that the seizures would at least decrease in number or severity.

I listened to his reassuring rejoinders and reasoned, *Yes, I can do this—I think. My seizures might end—it could be great.* Then I pictured the surgeon's blade near my skull and heard my father's voice the first time I'd mentioned the surgery option years earlier. *Brain surgery?? You don't want them messing with your brain! One false move, and it's all over*!

My mind vacillated between those thought streams like a battered ping pong ball.

An early riser by nature, I contemplated my dilemma in bed as morning light filled my room. Earlier that year we had added a dormer to our unfinished attic to create a master bedroom for Mark and me. Carpenters ripped the innards of our home's midpoint and threaded a large joist through the center of our two-family house to support the additional six hundred square feet. The job took six months.

I lay in my renovated room as sunlight filtered in, the walls freshly painted matching turquoise and teal, the wood floors shiny and new. Mere months ago, the space was a mishmash of crossbeams and unfinished walls, pink insulation hanging out and boxes of stuff strewn about.

I wavered for five weeks. Then I decided brain surgery could be a similar process to the attic renovation: a necessary onerous disruption that would result in long-term excellent outcomes. I was still scared, but Dr. R told me he'd performed more than fifteen hundred such operations. Dr. R was the innovator of temporal lobectomy—if anybody could safely pull it off, he was it. My decision made, with newfound enthusiasm, I reached out to Dr. R's assistant. I told them I would call them in January to schedule the operation for spring after I'd been at my new job a bit longer.

I informed friends and family about my decision and explained the risks continued seizures posed to my own long-term health and the challenges of raising the kids. Imagining a scenario where I'd have to defend my choice, and allay his anxiety, I expected my father to freak out, but he surprised me with his simple response: "I understand why you made this choice."

In January, I learned Dr. R was taking a leave of absence. I had determined him *the one* who could pull off the gruesome procedure and made peace with my fears. I was devastated that my plan wasn't an option. Dr. R's assistant gave me the name of a neurosurgeon in Boston and wished me luck. I'd never heard of the doctor and researching him felt like going back to square one. My best option had become Dr. A.

Over the winter, I met with two other Boston neurologists who gave reassuring second opinions about Dr. A's skills. My web surfing revealed that Dr. A had performed only about eighty temporal lobectomies, a figure that paled in comparison to the number performed by Dr. R.

One neurologist I consulted pointed out that the actual number of successful surgeries didn't matter—after a certain number of effective procedures, which he didn't quantify, a doctor was considered good, and Dr. A met the mark. The other neurologist gave her a ringing endorsement, claiming that if he had a family member who needed brain surgery, he would suggest they see Dr. A.

Pre-surgery consultations conjured visions of my head being sliced and diced.

"I feel slightly sick right now," I said to the consulting neurologist as he looked at the computer screen.

"It's an undertaking for sure," he acknowledged. "But try not to worry. I reviewed your medical history and the results of your pretests. Off the record, this operation is what we'd call a 'slam dunk' in my field."

Basketball players have the most control and highest success rate when they make slam dunks. I asked Dr. A to see she if had a surgery date available in late April.

❧ ☙

Three weeks before surgery, I had a Wada test. Named after the doctor who invented it, a Wada test confirms the dominant side of the brain. People's dominant brain side is typically the opposite of their dominant hand. As I'm right-handed, neurologists assumed my left hemisphere dominant. The Wada test would hopefully corroborate it, as Dr. A planned to cut a piece of the right side out. If not, surgery would be a no go.

Though the Wada test was less invasive than surgery, it was more intrusive than anything I'd ever done. In preparation, I received a four-page instruction sheet with logistics and descriptions of what to expect.

The Wada test is a triple-whammy: a magnetic resonance angiogram, where they examine the brain's blood vessels, followed by a consecutive barbiturate-dousing of each side of my brain, all the while recording results on an EEG. I was especially alarmed about the daunting technique doctors used to direct the barbiturates to the brain.

"Listen to this," I read to Mark the night before the test. "It says they inject a numbing medicine into my groin like the dentist does into my mouth when I get cavities filled."

I cringed, imagining needles stuck in my delicate gumline. "And before they soak my brain with barbiturates, they have to squirt dye into its vessels to outline the area and make sure there are no clots or anything in the way."

Envisioning that sharp poke to my crotch followed by a tube wedged inside scared me more than imagining barbiturates and purple pigment gushing into my head. "It says that the test isn't painful after they inject the numbing agent," I read out loud, my voice shaky.

Protocol required I go home accompanied from the Wada test, as I might still be sedated. I had to be at the hospital by 6:30 a.m., so Mark would take the kids to school and then meet me at the hospital.

74

"I'm glad you'll be there," I added. "I know you don't like to miss work." I felt a little guilty about the test impeding his work day. At least he'd been at his job almost a year, long enough to prove himself.

We sat on the red couch post children's bedtime. I lifted my feet onto the coffee table and leaned into the cushy pillows. While he would prefer never to miss work, Mark would not complain.

My gratitude was about more than the Wada test—there were multiple appointments leading up to the day of surgery, and more missed work days coming up with the surgery scheduled. As I pondered the alarming details of the Wada test, I also took heart in Mark's dedication—both to me and to the surgery.

I was scared and even skeptical about surgery's seventy percent success rate. Ever the optimist, Mark insisted that possible long-term positive outcomes outweighed the mediocre odds and certainly the inconvenience of missed workdays.

Sometimes, his optimism seemed unrealistic to me to the point of annoyance, but that night, his positive outlook helped me keep calm. As I lay in bed, I could relax a little. Just as the carpenter's pillar supported my renovated bedroom, Mark served as my truss, doing his best to support me through the Wada test and the surgery.

᯼ ᯽

I checked in to Boston's Brigham and Women's Hospital the next morning, signed release forms, changed into a hospital gown, and stashed my earrings in a pocket.

When the neuro-radiologist outlined the Wada test components, I still feared the needle near my crotch more than anything. He escorted me to the testing room, where they laid me down on a table beneath a special x-ray, hooked electrodes to my head, and surrounded the table with blue drapes, until only my head was exposed.

A perfect dark square outlined in white centered over my head, the x-ray machine suspended above me. I heard a faint beeping in the background. Every move I made was under scrutiny.

The radiologist shaved and sterilized my groin, the antiseptic cool against my delicate skin. "We're going to administer the numbing agent," he announced.

The dreaded moment. I employed my usual dentist's office tactic and squeezed my eyes shut as tightly as possible as I hoped the tension in my face could distract me from the needle's sharp point, mere inches from my genitals. The strategy was only ever half successful at the dentist's office, and that day was no different.

I inhaled sharply from the ache in the right side of my crotch. I felt some vague sensations in the vicinity as the doctor threaded a catheter inside me, and I knew from the prep talk that the catheter was being directed to an artery in my neck. Shortly after that, I sensed a sharp, weird taste in my mouth—that must be the contrast dye redirected to my brain. He instructed me to lie as still as possible. Meanwhile, the electrodes and the x-ray machine above my head recorded everything.

After some vague prodding in my groin—perhaps more dye directed through the catheter—the entire right side of my body went limp. They injected amobarbital, the barbiturate that would temporarily knock out half my brain. A few minutes later, they pulled the blue curtains back, and there were Dr. P and a team of practitioners hovering near my table.

"She's ready now," I heard one of them say.

I was on display, but too woozy to care. Dr. P showed me household items—a toothbrush, some tape—and juvenile picture cards with brightly colored objects—a cat, an apple. Moments later, Dr. P asked me what I had just seen. Although foggy from the anesthetic, I thought my recall near perfect. Dr. P wrapped up the show-and-tell game.

"Okay, we're going to wait a few minutes for the anesthetic to wear off," Dr. P announced. "When the right side of your brain is fully recovered, we'll put the left down."

After a respite, Dr. P pulled the blue curtains around my x-ray table, and I could feel them poking my leg as they adjusted the catheter. The second time, I wasn't shocked by the sharp taste in my mouth nor by the warm sensations in my face from the contrast dye. When Dr. P appeared with her stack of cards, I *thought* I was ready for the game. She showed me a series of bright pictures, waited a moment, and took out a card with an apple on it.

"Did you see this one before?" I remembered diddly squat. *Was that an apple or a bear before the train card?* I wasn't sure. *Damn, this is hard.*

"Yes," I replied, though I wasn't certain. Never indicating whether my answers were right or wrong, Dr. P kept a straight face as she introduced cards. But even under the dizzying effects of the anesthetic, I sensed I was failing. When Dr. P finished, I was relieved to be left alone.

The anesthetic wore off. The left side of my brain recovered, and Dr. P appeared to administer a final round of tests with her cards, which I sailed through. The radiologist opened the curtains, removed the electrodes from my head, and disconnected the catheter from my body, replacing it with a bandage over the small puncture. The procedure took about an hour.

The staff instructed me to stay in bed and wheeled me to a recovery room where Mark waited. I smiled weakly at him as he got up from the gray plastic chair next to the window.

"You're all set for now," the radiologist announced. "The nurses will be by to check the pulse in your legs and the dressing where the catheters were inserted."

"Can she go home today?" Mark asked eagerly.

"Probably in a few hours." She glanced up at the round white analog clock on the wall, which read 10:30. "Around 2:30," she declared. "The nurses need to be sure your circulation is back to normal," she added and exited the room. Mark approached the bed.

"It's over," I said, voicing my relief.

"Did it hurt?" he asked.

"Yes, about as much as I thought it would—far worse than the dentist," I said. "My leg is still a little sore under there." I picked up the hospital gown and pointed at the bandage on my inner right thigh. The location of the gauze patch—adjacent to my pubis—was enough to make Mark wince. "I'm glad it's over," I repeated. "I think I got the results I needed."

"What's that mean?"

"When they put the right side of my brain under, I could still remember everything. But when they put the left side down, I was lost. So the right side isn't doing much to support my memory skills, and I will probably still have recall abilities if they cut a piece out. Dr. P is going to get back to me to let me know."

"So, the brain surgery is likely going to happen soon?"

"By the end of the month, Dr. A said," and I noted, "I'm starving." I hadn't eaten since the night before per doctors' orders. I also wanted to avoid reminiscing about the surgery. "Can you get me some lunch, please? Something better than hospital food—to celebrate."

"Sure." Mark went to the Au Bon Pain in the hospital lobby, and promptly returned with a turkey avocado sandwich, which I devoured. About three hours later, after multiple rounds of pulse checks, the nurse said I could leave. The puncture spot was tender but on its way to healing.

A couple days later, Dr. P called and confirmed the analysis I shared with Mark. The left side of my brain was dominant. When the right side of my brain was down, I breezed through the tests. When the left side was down, I remembered zilch.

During the phone call, Dr. P also said she was ninety percent sure Dr. A was available to perform the operation on April 29.

Since the tests verified that the left side of my brain was so strong and capable, I should have taken comfort in the fact that the right side of my brain was somewhat expendable. That the surgery was possible meant freedom from seizures might be attainable—the prospect dangled before me, as hopeful and glittery as a disco ball.

But with the surgery prospect looming even larger, I was scared shitless.

Countdown to the Big Cutout

My father turned seventy in early April. As he was somewhat shy, Dad typically did not go for big birthday celebrations. But given the seven-decade milestone, his three adult children wouldn't let the day go unnoticed, so that year he agreed to a family party. The moderately sized gathering included my family, Greta's husband, Jeremy, and their children, Joyce, Richard, Daniel and his wife, Jenny, and my father and Chris. We gathered on a Saturday at Greta's home in the nearby Boston suburb of Natick.

The aroma of Jeremy's chili greeted us when we entered the yellow duplex through the dining room. The kids ran off to find their cousins upstairs. The granite kitchen countertop had the food set-up, so I placed the mushroom strata I'd baked amongst the fare. Mark and I left Greta and Jeremy to the last-minute table setting and joined the other adults in the living room. Dad, Jenny, and Daniel had settled on the purple couch across from Joyce, Richard, and Chris.

"Happy seventieth, Stanley," Mark said as we descended upon the remaining chair and ottoman. I saw Mark's polite reaching out for what it was —an attempt to toss kind celebratory words at my father despite their history of tensions over politics and parenting choices.

"Yeah, happy birthday," I chimed in, eager to keep their dialogue on neutral—even positive—territory for as long as possible. Their recurrent squabbles left me edgy, anticipating the next argumentative bomb while yearning for them to get along better.

"Thanks," Dad responded, rising briefly to shake Mark's hand and embrace me in a quick hug. Chris followed his lead and hugged me, speaking as she did.

"Laura, I heard your test went well," she said of the previous week's grueling Wada test. I had relayed the results to my father and asked that he share them with Chris. Though only nine days had passed, the Wada test felt like eons ago. I'd since firmed up the surgery date with Dr. A. I was in serious countdown mode—only seventeen days until they cut open my head.

"Yeah, the test found that my important memory functions are all on the left side, so it's safe to go ahead and slice and dice on the right," I said, trying to make light of the procedure. I suspected Chris felt extra anxious on my behalf. My downplay attempted to deflect her apprehension and conceal my fears.

"Yes, I heard from Stanley," Chris said. "So, April 29 is the day?"

Suddenly I realized everybody in the room was listening and that the day's gathering would be as much about me as about celebrating Dad's seventieth.

"That's right. It's the Tuesday after spring break, so the kids will be back in school."

"What kind of help will you need?" Joyce asked. "We might be able to watch the kids here and there."

"And they can come over here on the weekend after the surgery, if you want," Greta offered.

"Chris and I are coming down on that Tuesday to spend the night at your place," Dad said.

From there, the discussion turned into an all-hands-on-deck brainstorm. Greta offered to set up a Lotsa Helping Hands account for me, which Mark would use to update family and friends as well as to coordinate post-surgery visits and assistance. Daniel and Jenny offered to bring dinner over. I looked around the room, touched by the outpouring of familial support—maybe even a little surprised, given Dad and Chris's recent choice to move to Maine.

When Dad retired the previous year, he and Chris suddenly moved from western Massachusetts to Portland, Maine. Chris had Parkinson's, which was progressing, and Dad knew she would enjoy living near the beach. Massachusetts' coastal properties were out of their price range, so they found something in Maine. At the time, it confounded me that they'd chosen to move farther away from Greta's and my families, not closer. Over the years, Dad repeatedly spouted the fact that it took only thirty minutes of additional driving to their

Portland home. But that never allayed the disappointment I felt over their decision.

Over the years, I couldn't mask it, and I was glad when they moved back to Massachusetts in 2019. Thanks to the birthday celebration and pre-surgery planning, that day I put aside my discontent. When I looked around the room, I knew that—despite my perceptions of their emotional shortcomings—my family members had my back in their way. The reinforcement was heartening.

At seventy years old, Dad was only twenty-two years older than me, a difference that seems smaller and smaller the older I get. My father's once brown curly mop had turned all gray. Though his hairline had receded significantly, he still had a considerable amount of hair left. At sixty-six, Chris was even closer age wise, but the Parkinson's was taking its toll. Seated next to Dad, she looked elegant and sturdy in a flowy, olive-green tunic. But due to the Parkinson's, she was often shaky when she walked, a symptom that left her emotionally delicate.

I appreciated their presence a bit more.

"Time to celebrate the birthday boy," Greta announced a while later. She brought in a chocolate ganache cake and called upstairs to the kids. "It's time to wish Grandpa a happy birthday!"

We sang the birthday ditty, giving Dad his uncomfortable moment in the spotlight as he blew out the candle.

"Photo op!" Greta yelled. "Kids come gather around Grandpa so I can get a picture," she instructed, eager to document the event with a Facebook-worthy shot. She got Dad and the cake with the four grandchildren surrounding him.

Distracted by the matrix I was creating in my head, I absorbed the scene at surface level only. I was mapping out which sitters I would email to fill the childcare gaps my family couldn't cover. Of course, the matrix diverted me from what truly weighed on my mind: with no guarantee of a positive outcome, I was seventeen days away from having my brain carved up. Would I even be capable of creating such a matrix post surgery? Who knew? No matter how strong the family scaffolding, I wasn't sure how I was going to fare at the other end of the procedure.

✿ ✿

I operated on autopilot during the last days prior to surgery. At the time, I was consulting at an adult education program in South Boston, a position I'd held for eight months. My employer—I'll call it South Boston Education Center or SBEC—was affiliated with large Catholic institutions and operated by nuns. Staff knew I had epilepsy, and I'd discussed the upcoming surgery with my manager, Harvey. During April, I spent my time wrapping up loose ends with the intent of returning—perhaps even as a staff member—sometime after I recovered.

At home, I tried to prepare the children. Liam's guidance counselor suggested sharing minimal information about my brain surgery until a couple days before the operation.

"I think you want to keep it simple," Barry suggested. "Say something like 'Mommy's getting a cut in her head to make her feel better and hopefully to make the seizures stop.'"

"But what if they ask more questions? Liam almost certainly will."

"Then say something like, 'Those are details you don't need to know. Mom's doing this because she has seizures, which makes you worry about her, and kids shouldn't have to worry so much.'" I'd drawn my courage from that exact concern. Of course, the kids would also worry about the surgery, but I liked Barry's suggested language.

Though I'd been doing my best to take care of business and maintain a sense of normalcy, the upcoming operation seemed anything but normal. My brain knew it too. Within a day of my meeting with Barry, I had three complex partial seizures. Joyce noted that perhaps the seizure cluster constituted my brain's way of affirming the surgery decision, as if my brain were saying, *See, the surgery might bring an end to this situation. Go for it!* I thought anxiety about potential negative post-surgery outcomes triggered the seizures.

Two of the three seizures happened at the kids' school—one at drop-off, one at pickup. In the morning inside the building, I'd just had a brief visit to Liam's first grade classroom where parents had been invited to see their children's final art projects. I intended the classroom visit as a quick detour, since I had proposals to work on for SBEC.

My plan derailed when the seizure hit as I walked through the school's dim first-floor hallway. I really didn't remember much beyond the uncomfortable clutch in my belly. One minute I was in the hallway, and when I came out of the seizure, I was in the school nurse's office. *Somebody must have witnessed the seizure and brought me here. Who? Was Liam's teacher involved? Did she notice the seizure?* I saw the time—8:45. I hadn't been there very long.

Flustered and embarrassed, I explained to Nurse Liz, "I've got to get going. I'm okay, and I've got to get to work." All true words, but Nurse Liz's furrowed brow revealed her concern.

"You sure you're okay?"

"I'm fine," I pronounced. I gathered my belongings to head home, where I worked on a grant application. By the time I went to pick the kids up from school, I had submitted the application, caught up on emails, and contacted a potential new babysitter. As I waited in the schoolyard for the kids' dismissal, I wasn't thinking about the seizure I'd had earlier. But when pre-seizure belly twitching kicked in, I knew where my brain and body were at.

Oh no, not again! And in front of the teachers, parents and the kids to boot!

I don't remember much beyond the belly tingles—it's likely I twitched and paced in the schoolyard, but when I came out of the seizure, medics surrounded me, a gurney nearby.

Had they put me on that? I wondered.

I scanned the yard, searching for Liam and Amelia and processed the implications of what just happened. *Which parents saw that? What would they think of me now? What would the kids' friends think of me, or them?* I found the kids playing with friends on the playground structure. Engaged, they climbed up the brown ladder, their friend's mother Renée watching them from the bench.

Everybody had probably seen everything, I surmised. I turned my attention to the EMT by my side. "I'm feeling better now. I don't need to go to the hospital. I just want to go home."

"Are you certain you're okay?"

"Yes, I'm sure. Here, I can sign the papers for you," I said, eager to get rid of the medics. I was embarrassed on the kids' behalf—

now their friends had seen their mother out of sorts—doing who knows what?

After I signed the paperwork and sent the EMTs on their way, my cellphone rang, and I saw Mark's name flash across.

"Are you okay?" he asked when I picked up. "LeeAnne called me and said you'd had a seizure." Another schoolyard parent, LeeAnne had a son who played with Liam when they were younger. I knew LeeAnne tried to help but I felt self-conscious on the phone.

"Yeah, it happened here in the schoolyard. Somebody called the ambulance."

"So, you're okay?" Mark asked again.

"Yes, fine—really. Honestly, I'm not sure this seizure was any bigger than usual. I think staff felt they had to call 911, because I also had a seizure here at drop-off."

"You sound okay," he said, his voice tentative. "I am," I assured him. The sky had darkened with clouds. "It's about to rain. We're going straight home. I'll be fine." I gathered Liam and Amelia and skulked away from the schoolyard toward our house.

The children were subdued.

"That must have been scary," I said. "I'm so sorry."

"Yeah—I was playing on the tot lot, and then the ambulance was there," Amelia said. "All my friends got scared and ran to the basketball court." The court was behind the school, away from the playground area.

"Jeanie ran over when she saw you have the seizure and made LeeAnne call 911," Liam added. The dreaded lunch aide Jeanie apparently groused as she served up food. Yet, she kicked into red alert and tried to help that day. Perhaps the kids would view her through a new lens.

"I'm really sorry," I repeated. What else could I say? "I'm okay now, I promise," which was true. The situation's implications rattled me, but as we walked home, the post-seizure hazy phase had passed.

"And I'm going to take some steps to try to get these seizures to stop—I promise," I told the children. Recalling Barry's advice, I kept the statement vague. The surgery date was still over two weeks away.

"What steps?" Liam asked. Although I didn't know for certain the seizures would stop, I borrowed a page from Mark's optimistic playbook. I could vow that I was taking action steps.

"I'm going to the doctors at the end of the month. They're going to try to help me. I think they can now."

The kids took that in as we walked the last block home.

"Do you want to make popsicles?" I asked as we entered the house. I needed to redirect our attention to something more pleasant.

"Yeah!" Amelia took the bait. "Can we make them strawberry flavored?"

"Sure. Lemme text Dad, and then we'll get started."

Home now. About to make popsicles with kids. Feeling fine.

I hit send and got to work blending frozen berries, ripe bananas, and yogurt in the food processor. I filled the silver popsicle holders with pink viscous goo while the kids threaded round metal tops with popsicle sticks and popped them on. The project served as the perfect distraction. Then my cellphone rang, the school's number flashing across it. *Uh oh.*

"This is Laura," I said, my voice as cool and collected as I could keep it.

"Laura, it's Barry. I wanted to make sure you're alright."

"Yes, I'm fine. The kids and I are making popsicles. Mark will be home in about an hour," I added.

"Good, I'm glad you're okay. Listen, Principal Davis wants to meet with you. She's concerned about the episodes at school today and wants to know what you intend to do."

Barry's words infuriated me. He knew full well what I was about to do—we'd discussed it that week.

"Did you tell her I'm having brain surgery at the end of this month?" I snapped at him.

"No, I didn't disclose that. You can tell her when you meet with her if you want."

We scheduled the meeting for Tuesday, and I fretted all weekend. The school's staff had witnessed too much, and Mrs. Davis was concerned about the kids' safety. Would she feel compelled to call outside authorities? It wasn't the only time I'd had two seizures in one day around the children—just the first time it happened at their school.

At least the surgery date was in place. If the principal was having thoughts about calling child protective services, my scheduled temporal lobectomy provided a strong card to play.

The principal greeted Mark and me promptly on Tuesday morning, and shuttled us into the conference room, where the school nurse and the vice-principal joined us. Known entities sat at the table. Principal Davis was friendly, personable, and generally well-liked amongst parents. In my experience, her second-in-command Ms. Baker was the hard-liner when it came to student discipline. I'd had the fewest dealings with Nurse Liz, but her kind, nurturing demeanor matched what I would expect from a pediatric nurse practitioner.

Mark and I sat on one side of the table, across from the others. Waiting for Principal Davis to lead the conversation, I twirled my hair nervously.

"Thank you both for coming in today. We're glad to see you're feeling better, but we're concerned about the episodes you had at school on Friday. They looked significant. It seems like the children might be at risk when they happen. What's your plan?"

What's my plan? I was so outraged by her callous question I momentarily forgot the obvious answer.

"I could stay off your campus, but short of that, I can't guarantee this won't happen again. I don't *plan* my seizures—they just happen."

I looked at Nurse Liz and silently implored her to back me up with medical facts, which she did. Principal Davis acknowledged that banning me from the school was not a good option. Perhaps she wished she could, but we both knew that would be illegal.

"Actually, Laura is scheduled to have brain surgery, which will hopefully stop her seizures," Mark piped up.

Oh right, there is a plan!

Relief swept over me as Mark steered the conversation away from my prickly response and toward the scheduled action step. Happy to let him take over, I sighed as all three of them turned their eyes on Mark.

"When is that happening?" Principal Davis asked.

"April 29—two weeks from today. Laura will be in the hospital about four days. We have friends and family helping us look after the kids that week. Full recovery will take about eight weeks, and there's a really good chance she'll have no—or at least fewer—seizures."

Mark put the most positive spin possible on the surgery—something I couldn't do. I relaxed a bit as I listened to the exchange. Clearly, the assurance was enough for the principal.

An active parent at the kids' school, I volunteered in multiple capacities and attended my kids' activities. Although after that day I never had another seizure at the school, I imagined some parents and teachers remembered the seizures and thought of me as the *mom who has seizures*.

I also wondered what biases administrative staff held about me. When Principal Davis retired about a year after my surgery, I joined the small goodbye gathering attended by many parents. Everybody bid her a happy farewell and asked what would come next.

"Yeah, what's your plan?" I called out from my cafeteria seat as I recalled that dreadful meeting. I didn't care much about Mrs. Davis's retirement activities. I was happy to see her leave, as that would be one less person who knew about my health condition. But it sure felt good to lob the line back in her face, although I doubt she caught my reference.

Elective Slice and Dice

The week prior to brain surgery was the kids' school spring break, so I spent extra time lining up the additional childcare required to cover my work hours. Multiple times, I had to craft and reconfigure the babysitter matrix—comprised of my part-time hours and available time of revolving college students I hired to watch the kids. Maintaining it was a complicated unpaid job, so I was flying high when I had the matrix configured for spring break. Then Dr. P called.

"Dr. A said your MRI images from last week weren't as sharp as she'd like. She'd like you to do another one."

You've got to be friggin' kidding, right? I thought. *My perfected matrix is out the window?*

"You can call the main number to get an appointment. I sent the order, so they'll know it's time sensitive."

Nope, she's not kidding. Well, if the brain surgeon thinks she needs clearer results, I'd better make sure she gets them. I scheduled the additional MRI exactly a week before surgery.

On top of managing work, childcare arrangements, and dealing with the school principal, I endeavored to keep calm and mentally prepare for surgery. Inevitably, my mind fell back on my biggest fears: *What if this doesn't work? What if I lose my memory? What if my personality is altered in some way?*

Mark reminded me of all the pre-testing results, which indicated the operation would likely be successful. As my partner, he was my first go-to person, and he provided a different deeper level of support than any doctor could. Yet, just like the doctors' words, Mark's assurances fell short. They couldn't really address my grief—I was heartsick that the chaotic neurons in my head could be controlled only by mutilation. I felt I had failed in some way.

Perhaps if I had mastered the relaxation exercises I'd tried years before, I might have completely stopped the seizures using meditation techniques. If only my brain had been a little "better behaved," I might have responded to one of the seventeen anti-epileptic drugs I'd tried over the decades.

Each time I fell into that pit of negative ruminations, I gently pulled myself out by issuing a soothing reminder: *I was not at fault or bad.* Although brain surgery felt like an extreme option, I'd done my research and had determined it as the path to take. I had confidence in the decision. Rather than on the crappy what-ifs, I tried to focus on the ultimate outcome I hoped for—a possible end to seizures. I also promised to take care of my brain—of my whole body—to foster a quick recovery by comforting myself with forgiving reflections and soothing images of a speedy healing process, one that involved making peace with my grief and guilt.

My parents didn't raise us religiously, so praying to a god wasn't an option for me. I've always believed that if there truly was a benign deity looking over me, I wouldn't have been saddled with refractory seizures in the first place. Two friends recommended a book, *Prepare for Surgery, Heal Faster • A Guide of Mind-Body Techniques*, which came with a relaxation CD. Although meditation practice hadn't stopped my seizures, I was desperate for comfort and courage, so I pored through the book's pages as I lapped up the author's advice.

I calmed myself with the relaxation exercises. I attempted to turn my worries into soothing energy, generating my own healing images. Four days before the operation, I sent my closest friends and family an email asking them to think of me on surgery day:

Next Tuesday I'm checking in to Brigham and Women's Hospital around 5:30AM, and at around 7:30, they will begin administering an anesthetic. The neurosurgeon begins the actual business of slicing and cutting at 8:30, and the operation is five to six hours long! Needless to say, I'm scared. I'm most scared I'll go through this process, and still have seizures. I'm asking friends to think about me at 7:15 on Tuesday morning, and send your love, good wishes, and support my way, which I will receive in the hospital in the shape of a teal colored blanket of love. (If you're not sure how to do this, recall a time we spent together, where you felt we truly connected. When you remember that time, as if I was right there with you, wrap me in the teal blanket of love, beginning at 7:15AM.) Thanks to everybody for your support.

I sent the email out via the Lotsa Helping Hands site Greta set up for me. Then I read the statements I'd written. The book suggested saying them aloud before and during surgery, as the body is most suggestible then. Clearly, I wasn't going to say anything to myself during a temporal lobectomy, so I read the words multiple times in the days leading up to surgery day, and brought the statements to the hospital, to review when I woke up:

1. Following this operation, you will feel comfortable, and you will heal very well.
2. Your operation has gone very well.
3. Following this operation, you will be hungry for fresh lemonade. You will be thirsty and able to drink easily.
4. Following the operation, you will rest and relax as long and as much as you need to heal and regain your energy.

Something I read about the surgery inspired the third statement. I knew they'd insert a breathing tube down my throat, and I'd wake up extra thirsty. Homemade lemonade is one of my indulgences. I regularly keep lemons on hand, so there's often a jar of my lemonade in the fridge. I didn't really expect fresh lemonade upon waking, but the vision comforted me.

❧ ☙

While I grappled with my fears and internal bugaboos, Mark managed the hellish domestic logistics. By April 29, Mark had lined up people to check in on me and sitters/friends to help watch the kids for the two weeks following surgery. My father and Chris would pick the kids up from school in the early afternoon and stay at our house for a few days. The night before surgery, my buddy Rich and his wife, Sophie, arrived at our house with their dog Dreamgirl.

Rich was my oldest friend in town—we'd been roommates with a myriad of other friends at three different addresses over the decades. I called him and Sophie the kids' fruncle andfrauntie." Another Jewish New Yorker from the Bronx, Rich shared memories, friends,

90

and experiences with me from the six years we'd roomed together, but we'd always been just buddies. We'd seen each other through breakups and romances and participated in each other's wedding ceremonies. Rich had been with me during several of the few grand mal seizures I'd had during adulthood.

I wanted Rich's family in our home on that penultimate day because I knew they would bring a sense of levity that none of us was capable of. Mark and I focused too much on the surgery to pay good attention to the kids. I suspected that when the grandparents watched them after school, they wouldn't conceal their anxiety while the children played.

I smiled when I heard Rich call from the bottom of the front stairwell followed by the quick rat-a-tat-tat of Dreamgirl's paws, as she bounded upstairs toward the living room.

"They're here," I called to the kids. "Dreamgirl, too."

Clutching their overnight bags, Rich and Sophie clamored in as the kids gathered around their white shaggy mutt, happily petting her coat.

"Ta da! We're here!" Rich stretched his arms wide to give and receive hello hugs and then briefly joined the dog petting fest. "Dreamgirl's hungry," he stated, rifling through his bag for some dog food.

"Who wants to help feed her?" asked Sophie, another curly girl with untamed dark tresses.

"I do," Liam asserted.

"Yeah. Me, too!" Amelia chimed in.

"Oh, good. Dreamgirl will get her dinner extra quickly tonight. She'll be happy," Sophie said.

Relief washed over me as the kids scampered to the kitchen behind my friends. I watched them prepare the food. They carefully helped Rich scoop viscous mush into the silver bowl. As Dreamgirl eagerly approached her meal, the kids beamed, and I knew we'd all make it through the next morning fine despite the weight of what lay ahead.

After dinner we did our best to keep the evening as normal as possible. Stories and toothbrushing followed, and the adults gathered near the kids' beds for final goodnight hugs.

"You remember that tomorrow Mom and Dad are leaving for Mom's surgery at the hospital before you wake up," I said. "Rich and Sophie will get you ready for school."

"When will you be home?" Liam asked.

"Hopefully on Thursday. The doctor said they keep you in the hospital for two days. Grammy Christina and Papa Stanley are coming from Portland to stay for a couple days. They'll pick you up at school tomorrow. Dana will also be around for a little while to help out."

We'd lined up a sitter for the first afternoon. Mark had sent the grandparents a long email with bullet-pointed instructions on how to navigate the house and an outline of the kids' daily routines.

"I'm going to miss you," Amelia said.

"Yes, of course. That's why all these friends and family are coming to keep you company and take care of you."

"Let's have a group hug to wish your mom well and to comfort ourselves," Sophie suggested. Though I didn't have as long or tight a history with her as with Rich, we'd developed a close connection over time. Sophie was touchy-feely by nature, occasionally to an extreme by my standards, but that night I appreciated her unrestrained compassion. I snuggled Amelia on my lap with Liam next to me on one side, Mark on the other, as we crowded on the double bed in a sloppy group embrace.

"There. That was good," Rich pronounced, his enthusiasm contagious.

"I love you all," I said.

They'd be okay the next morning, and after school they'd have their grandparents with them. Now I had to focus on myself.

The adults gathered in the living room. It was only 9:15, and we'd planned an early bedtime for all. "Thanks for coming tonight," I said. "I'm so glad you'll be here with the kids in the morning."

"They seemed fine," Sophie observed.

"Yeah. We only told them the details of Laura's procedure over the weekend. We expected them to be anxious, but excitement over the prospect of Laura's seizures ending seemed to outweigh any anxiety they have about the operation" Mark noted.

"Yeah, at this point, it's really me who's the most freaked out," I said.

"Understandable," Rich said.

"Yes. Here, one more group hug, then bedtime," I suggested.

With Rich on my left, Mark on my right, and Sophie across from me, I reached my arms wide and bent my head in toward theirs, my eyes closed.

Lean now and take in this support while you can, I thought. *Memorize this moment so you can recall it tomorrow.*

Fortified by the gesture, I was ready to step back. "Good night," I said.

Upstairs in my room, I gathered essentials including my healing statements and a meditation CD into an overnight bag,.

This was it. Tomorrow Dr. A would be slicing into my head, taking out that "bad" part of my brain.

I was still more afraid of a screw-up than the pain. All the what-ifs collected in my head and weighed on me again: Memory loss. Personality change. Continued seizures despite all this effort.

"I'm scared," I said to Mark, who had joined me.

"Yes, of course. This is scary. But remember all the tests you took and the results showing this will likely work out well. That doctor called the operation a slam dunk, right?"

Mark's optimism was a double-edged sword, minimizing my fears and balancing my doubtful side. His optimism was critical to me. Speaking as an innate pessimist, I assume only a true optimist would agree to co-parent with a person who has epilepsy.

That night Mark's attempt to assuage my apprehension failed.

Right. Easy for him to say—nobody was taking a scalpel to his head. I smiled weakly.

"Here, come to bed," Mark said, patting my side of the bed. "We need to get to sleep early."

I followed Mark's directive and, leaning against the headboard as he draped his arm across my shoulders, I sat down next to him. I focused on the weight of his arm and the board supporting my back. *Lean into it,* I silently instructed myself again, as I nestled against Mark. *Remember the possible critical outcome: seizure control.* I meditated on it, steering my thoughts away from everything scary about the next day.

Mark dropped his arm over my shoulder and pulled me closer in. "You ready to go to sleep? We should turn in early."

"I need to read first." If I turned off the light at that moment, I wouldn't stop thinking about tomorrow. "Give me a piece of the Sunday *Globe*," I said.

I found a vaguely noteworthy article on powdered alcohol and read on until my lids felt heavy. About two thirds of the way through the piece, I felt myself conking out.

"Here," I said rousing myself just enough to hand the paper back to Mark and turn off my light. "G'night."

❧ ☙

The next morning, we arrived at 5:30 a.m. and were directed to the basement for check-in. Although based on written instructions, I expected it, but I was still struck by the dingy environs. I had imagined a bright room with daylight streaming through big windows. The dim room had beige shades pulled closed over high windows.

How will they see what they're doing?

A few minutes later, the nurse on duty came in with a thick stack of papers. "I'm Maddie," she said. I'm going to help you with your pre-procedure workups. Can you tell me your name, date of birth, and what you're here for?"

I gathered the quizzing was standard protocol, but it felt dumb. I was there to get the bad piece of my brain removed—they knew that. *Whatever . . .*

"I'm here for a right temporal lobectomy," I said.

"Good. Now can you tell me today's date and who the current president is?"

"April 29, 2014. Barack Obama."

"Good. I'm going to take your vital signs after you change into this johnny. Then I'll insert an IV into your arm. It will stay there through the procedure, and you'll be ready to be taken up to neurosurgery."

An upper floor would surely be brighter than this. Phew! My relief negated any anxiety over the IV insertion. And when Maddie efficiently strapped a blue rubber strip over my bicep and inserted the IV with minimal discomfort, her proficiency assured me.

"Okay, you're all set for Dr. A now. They'll come fetch you when she's ready," Maddie said. While I appreciated her skills, her cheery demeanor didn't suit the occasion.

Then the waiting began. The surgery was scheduled for 9:00— an hour and a half away. Mark and I quietly sat in the dark check-in room together. When scary thoughts and what-ifs crept into my head, I pushed them away by reading my healing statements. I distracted myself by skimming the news online. In that bed, IV in arm, I just wanted to get the damned thing over with.

Thanks to operating room preparations, the anesthesiologist didn't come down to get me until nearly ten. He explained the effects of the anesthetic.

"I'm going to inject it through the IV in your arm, and it will kick in quickly. I'll ask you to count backwards from a hundred, and you'll be under long before you get to one," he explained. "Any questions?"

Let's just get this done. "Are you doing this now?" I asked.

"I'll bring you up to the operating room first. Are you ready?"

I looked at Mark, who'd been listening from the wooden hospital chair. Typical Mark, he seemed calm. I might have been freaking out a little if he were the one about to have brain surgery, but not him. He walked over to the side of my bed and took my hand.

"Yes," I answered. Mark bent over and pecked me on the cheek.

"Good luck, Sweetie," he said, his voice quiet.

And then it was time. They wheeled me to an elevator and through a maze of halls to a large room lit by multiple harsh overhead fluorescent bulbs. They transferred me to the operating table as Dr. A entered the room. She wore blue scrubs and a light blue surgical cap, which resembled an unglamorous shower cap, over her hair.

This was it: Dr. A was about to cut my head open.

Forget the what-ifs. Replace them with that healing statement: Your operation will go well. Seizure-freedom at the other end. I took a deep breath and exhaled.

"We're going to administer the anesthesia now," the anesthesiologist informed me.

I felt a pinch in my arm, as the fluid dripped in. "Now count backwards from a hundred. Try to focus just on the numbers."

Pushing away the thoughts of a scalpel next to my brain, I followed his instructions. I was under around ninety-six and knocked out for the entire procedure, but I know roughly what happened from conversations I'd had with Dr. A and the online descriptions I'd read about temporal lobectomies. Based on them, the surgery went something like this: once I was anesthetized, they shaved the right side of my head and secured it in a skull-fixation device. Then Dr. A cut into my head—first the skin, revealing my skull, and next the skull itself.

And my brain was exposed. Dr. A performed electrical testing on neural pathways to reveal exactly where that mischievous bad spot was, and boom! Using her scalpel, scissors, and expertise, she extracted a kiwi-sized portion of brain tissue. I didn't feel or recall a thing.

I woke up several hours later with new brain architecture and questions. *Am I still me? Did brain reconstruction alter my personality?*

I took stock: I was back in a dimly lit hospital room with faint beeping in the background. I was woozy—my head felt too big for my body. Most significantly, though, I felt like myself. There was a tender spot on my left arm where an IV pierced my inner elbow. Later, I learned that it dripped pain killer into my body, which is probably how I could focus on lighting before I noticed the dull throb in my head. The pain was evident but not overpowering if I kept still.

When Mark walked in, I could easily focus on his tentative smile.

"You're up," he said, approaching the bed. He looked tired. Later, I read detailed mid-surgery email updates Mark sent my family and friends to apprise them of my status.

His words made me grateful I'd married an articulate patient writer.

"Yes. I made it. What time is it?"

"Six o'clock. You've been out for about eight hours."

Eight hours gone in the blink of an eye with a blade to my head. Yikes.

"How you feeling?"

"Not so bad, given the day I just had." My head was sore, but I had expected more pain. The ache in my head felt no worse than when I came out of a grand mal seizure.

"I spoke with Dr. A about an hour ago. She said the surgery went well. They knew exactly where to cut from the tests they did during the surgery. She was so sure they were spot on that they didn't run a second MRI after the surgery."

That sounded positive. I wanted to ask about the likelihood of seizures, but then a nurse walked in. Maddie had been replaced by the night-shift nurse, who introduced herself as Phyllis.

"Good to see you're up. They say the surgery went well. You're in the ICU, and for the first twenty-four hours, we need to examine you every thirty minutes to make sure your brain is stable. Let me see you wiggle your toes."

I followed her instructions, relieved to find it easy.

"Now follow my fingertip with your eyes, but don't move your head."

Again, no problem.

"And tell me the year and the president's name."

"2014. Barack Obama."

Pride and validation welled inside as I responded to Phyllis the first time—the tests further proved that I was still really me despite the missing chunk of brain tissue. By the third time, I found the drill annoying and exasperating when they woke me up multiple times in the middle of the night. By then, I rolled my eyes as I tossed out the year and Obama's name before Phyllis even asked.

They kept me in ICU through the next day, and I dozed on and off between the predictable quizzes. My head hurt with swelling around the U-shaped incision extending to my right eye, but exhaustion crushed me more than pain.

The next day, they let me eat a tiny bit, chewing only on the left side of my mouth. The bland applesauce made a pleasant distraction. Shortly after my snacking, Dr. A came to visit. She wore her scrubs and smiled as she approached my hospital bed. I was grateful to see her and eager to ask questions about the long-term outlook on seizure control.

"You're doing well," Dr. A declared, as she skimmed the nurses' records. "There were no complications during the surgery. We removed a piece of the right temporal lobe where there appeared to be misfiring neurons."

"So, does that mean the seizures will stop?" I asked.

"The outlook is good, but I can't say for certain that you'll never have seizures again."

Although her words weren't surprising, my face fell when I heard them.

"Our immediate goal is to keep you seizure-free during this initial recovery phase. Your brain is in the most fragile state it's ever been. Having a seizure now could impair its healing. You've had no seizure activity since yesterday, which is a great sign, but it's not a guarantee you won't have seizures again.

"As your brain heals from the surgery," she continued, "ideally it will adjust to its new configuration, and you'll hopefully remain seizure-free."

I yearned for a clear correlation between initial positive outcome and long-term outlook. I knew it was a case of magical thinking, yet Dr. A's words felt like a blow. That an eight-hour brain surgery couldn't provide a guarantee seemed unfair.

"I'm going to suggest they move you out of ICU, and I'll check in on you again later," she added. Then she left.

Dr. A had always said the odds of full seizure control were only seventy percent. I didn't really expect her to provide the reassurances I wanted, but I was still disappointed. After the day I'd just had, the pain in my skull, and the scar on my head, I wanted more.

Like a competitive sprinter who just raced in the heat, I deserved a dunk in the pond to cool down. But the water had dried up. Given that he always sees the glass as half full, I wasn't surprised by Mark's next words.

"You're getting out of the ICU later—that's great. And you've been seizure-free since the surgery. You're on your way," he added.

Yeah, but there were no guarantees. I didn't voice it aloud. I knew Mark's likely subsequent attempt to buoy my spirits wouldn't work, and I didn't want to hear it.

"Can you look in my backpack for me? I want to read those healing statements again."

Mark handed off the paper, and I skimmed the page as I focused on the two most relevant statements. *Your operation has gone very well.*

Yes, the nurses and Dr. A had all said that multiple times. I reread the line a couple more times. Then, *following this operation, you will feel comfortable, and you will heal very well.*

Hmm—no, I didn't feel comfortable. The spot where the IV stuck into my arm felt tender. I felt like I was lurching on a roller coaster thanks to painkillers swamping my brain. And the shaven area surrounding the suture-laced incision on my head was exposed and sore.

I nevertheless resolved to continue healing very well. Looking over my shoulder, Mark stood next to the hospital bed.

"I'm not feeling very comfortable, but I have to believe I'll heal," I told him.

"Yes, and we know you got statement two covered. Dr. A said the surgery was a success."

"Yes," I agreed.

Call the glass half full. I had made it through surgery with the important parts of my brain still intact. Side effects of surgery would likely abate before too long.

Later that day, following me with a liquid bag of electrolytes connected to my arm with an IV, the nurse helped me walk the hospital halls for the first time. I'd been lying down for well over twenty-four hours, so bearing weight felt strange. I welcomed nurse Phyllis's steady arm as I timidly shuffled to the end of the hall.

"Okay, let's turn around," Phyllis said, pivoting around to reorient us. By the time we traversed the corridor again, I had the hang of my stride.

Later I talked to the children on the telephone.

"Hi, Mom. Are you okay?" Liam asked, his words rushed and anxious.

"I am. My head still hurts, but I'm okay."

"Good. When are you coming home?"

"I'm not sure–maybe tomorrow."

"Good. Here's Amelia."

Liam handed the phone off to her, and we had a similarly short check in. Their sweet youthful voices lifted my spirits, but I suspected the truncated conversations signified their stress. Once again, they had to be brave.

I felt a pang of guilt.

❧ ❧

The hospital released me on Thursday afternoon less than forty-eight hours since the surgery ended. I'd assumed they'd want to keep watch for longer, and make sure my brain was stable. Instead, they increased my anti-epileptic drugs, AEDs, and sent me home with a bandage over my sutured skull, my remaining hair restrained in braids, and a bottle of opioid painkiller to mitigate my aching head. Although I was pleased and nervous to be going home, I wondered, *Is this too soon? What if I have a seizure?* I dwelled on it as I gingerly followed Mark up the front steps of our apartment. The kids—who had been playing at the table with my father and Chris—scrambled toward me.

"Mommy, you're home," Amelia said, hugging my legs.

"Mommy, you're okay!" Liam declared, following suit with his sister.

I placed my arms on each of their backs and traced my hands along their spines. As I basked in the warm greeting, my anxiety dissipated a little. I sat on the edge of the couch so I could see them better and extended my arms in their direction.

"Yes, I'm back, and I'm okay. Come here," I said, drawing them close in an unwieldy three-way hug. Amelia scooched next to me, and Liam planted himself solidly in front. I treasured the feel of them against me and inhaled the vaguely floral scent of their shampoo.

Mark appeared from the kitchen and handed me a glass of lemonade. "Here, I made this for you."

I was home. I redirected my thought from seizure fear to seizure freedom. After reviewing my previous fourteen years of seizure records, I determined that the longest I'd gone without having a complex partial seizure was thirty-five days back in 2011. On the calendar, I marked the following June 4, which would be the thirty-sixth day post surgery. My eyes on that prize, I opened the Lotsa Helping Hands site on my computer. I wanted to share my goal with family and friends, but before I could tap out the words, I read the update emails Mark sent while I was in the hospital. Mark posted six times over two days, the first update written when I was mid surgery.

All is going according to plan in operating room now, reports a nurse who phoned me. Surgery began about an hour late to ensure all preparations had been done completely. They're removing a kiwi-fruit-sized piece of brain tissue from above and in front of right ear so she will have to grow some of those beautiful curls back in due time! Nurse is supposed to call with another update around 3:15. I'll try to post another update afterward.

Less than two hours later, Mark informed everybody the doctor was patching up my head, and he posted when it was all over:

Neurosurgeon just briefed me in waiting room and surgery went well with no complications or surprises. They removed the brain tissue they targeted plus a tiny bit more. They were confident they removed what they needed. While it's great that surgery went smoothly, the surgeon can't offer any more clarity than she could prior to surgery on the likelihood that the procedure will provide long-term seizure control or reduction. It will take months to see how brain adapts to this new structure with a piece missing.

The following day, Mark updated everybody multiple times as I awakened and later gained abilities to eat and walk.

Mark's postings left me grateful I married a writer with the ability to describe what I'd undergone. Mark's consideration touched me as he took the time to keep my friends and family apprised. I also felt agitated again when I read the lack of clarity in Dr. A's long-term prognosis. Somehow, seeing it posted in Mark's careful words underscored the fragility of my brain *and* my circumstance. While the surgery was behind me, there was no guarantee it would have the effect I wanted. I'd crested the top of a steep hill only to find the beautiful view obfuscated by fog and clouds.

I needed to buoy my spirits and hope for the best. I noted my healing statements weren't focused on the long-term outlook. *What if*

I went through this only to have seizures anyway? No, this is not the time for gloom and doom. Stay focused on the goal: seizure freedom, if only one day at time for now.

Then I banged out my own email via the Lotsa Helping Hands list.

Thanks for your thoughts and good wishes. As you know, my surgery took place last Tuesday; it was about eight hours long. I'm still tired, and I'll probably be fatigued for about two weeks, but happily the worst is over! I'm typing this email, so I'm lucid enough to formulate these thoughts. The good news is that the pain is largely gone despite the 6-inch, U-shaped line of heavy-duty sutures in my head. Even better news than that is that I haven't any seizure activity since the surgery.

It's too soon to say that I won't ever have them again, but this positive beginning is a good sign. The neurosurgeon also said that, when they were doing the actual cutting and slicing, they could tell that the piece of my brain they cut away was indeed causing neurons to misfire, which is what causes seizures in the first place. So, while there are no guarantees, I'm somewhat optimistic. I'm asking you to wish for the long-term positive outcome of seizure freedom, which would have immeasurable positive life ramifications for me and my family.

Next Friday I have an appointment with the neurosurgeon, and if she says the sutures look like they're healing, she'll remove them from my head. The sutures look bizarre, and I'm not used to the punk shaven look on the right side of my head. But so be it. Thanks again for your well wishes.

I proofread my note and felt glad that it sounded more upbeat than the dark thoughts I was mired in only moments earlier. I hit send. Responses from near and far came in within hours.

"Yayayay! I am beyond elated, Laura. YOU DID IT," my longtime buddy and former MEDUSA colleague Robin wrote. "I am so proud of you and your family! Here's to a VERY HOPEFUL outcome! woo-hoo! Wear that punk hairdo in style, girlfriend—you have so earned it!"

❧ ❧

Two weeks post surgery, I met Dr. A for suture removal, and she advised me to taper off the painkillers. I'd been taking them four times daily, so I was happy to follow her advice. The opioids had caused me to feel dissociated, like I was watching my life in a movie. I replaced them with ibuprofen within three days. My head hurt more, but I preferred the increased pain to feeling sluggish and disconnected.

The day after the sutures came out, I freed my remaining hair from the braids, and my asymmetrical mop was a frizzy thick mess on the left. The shaven right side looked freaky with the U-shaped scar running from my temple over my ear. But once I washed my mane, my lopsided do returned to its abundantly curly state, and with my hair down, I couldn't even see the scar! I felt like crap, but my spirits soared at my normal looking image in the mirror.

Over the following weeks, I marveled over my speedy recovery. I had typical symptoms of ongoing slight fatigue and an ever-present mild headache, so I moved more slowly. I left the lifting and laundry to others, but life marched on, and I participated. When Amelia turned five in May, we organized a piñata fiesta for her.

Originally scheduled for the local playground, the party fell on a rainy day, so we had to invite guests to our home. My stepmother-in-law was staying with us for a week or so to help around the house while I recovered. Ruth and I had prepared a maraca-making crafts activity. We bought a case of six-ounce water bottles and some rice. Leading up to the party, we emptied the bottles, then covered them with gauzy medical tape and filled them with rice.

When the guests arrived, they found the bottles set out on the table with magic markers and other art supplies. Most of the parents didn't know about my surgery, and with the help of a scrunchie and a couple of bobby pins, there were no signs of scars on my shaven head. I chatted with guests and helped facilitate the crafts activity and later piñata, pizza, and cake.

The same week, I reached out to my manager, the director at SBEC, to restate my interest in returning there after I recovered. Some staff—including my manager, Harvey—had seen me have seizures, so I'd been up front with them about my surgery. I emailed with Harvey through May and learned that SBEC planned to establish full-time development positions in the fall. Harvey knew I didn't want to work full time and suggested I could work as a consultant though not on staff again in July if I felt up to it. Despite their ambiguity, the exchanges pleased me. Staff searches could take a while, so they might need a consultant well into August. Surely, I'd be better by then.

In early June, we went out to dinner to celebrate my thirty-six-day, seizure-free milestone. I felt up to walking the near-mile distance to the Flatbread Pizza restaurant in Davis Square. I savored the warm spring air, and the festive street musicians in the plaza on the way. Over dinner, Mark raised a wine glass in a toast. "To thirty-six days free of seizures and years more to come," he said. The kids and I lifted our lemonades in response, and we all clinked glasses.

Yes, this could be it—no more seizures ever. "Hear, hear," I chimed in.

To others in the restaurant, we looked like a family out for dinner on a weekend night. The kids engaged in siblings' taunts and giggles. But we were also acknowledging a milepost. It had been years since I'd gone more than a month without having a seizure. The milestone was evidence that the surgery *could* be the beginning of a seizure-free trend. I cautiously embraced the delightful possibility that buoyed my spirits that night.

The Unexpected Second Time

Once I made it past Day 36, I counted down to June 28, sixty days post surgery. On that day, I could go back to my regular workout regimen of thirty minutes on my exercise equipment. Given that I love to eat and have a muscular, somewhat zaftig physique, I find regular exercise critical.

I store the exercise machines in the corner of our master bedroom and use them about four times a week. I woke on June 28 eager to resume my routine of stretches followed by sessions on the stationary bike and elliptical machine. I huffed and puffed my way through, and by the end, I felt very sweaty and a little worn out but not especially sore or fatigued. More than anything, I was elated by accomplishment— I had succeeded at my post-surgery workout.

Later, while scrolling through emails at my desk, I noticed an odd misalignment of my fingers on the keyboard. My fingertips felt a tiny bit off from where they should rest on the letters. I lifted my hands off my desk and realigned my fingers on the keyboard. A moment later, they felt askew again. *This is weird.* Looking back, I recognize that strange physiological disarray as my first warning of what the day held. But at the time, I thought something was wrong with the keyboard, and I asked Liam if he'd adjusted it.

"No. Why would I do that?" he asked. Liam was right—my theory made no sense.

Rich had some carpentry work in our vicinity the day before and had slept over after a post-work visit with our family. Over breakfast we firmed our morning plan. We were all going to the mall, Assembly Row, to run errands.

We parked the car in the sprawling lot at the mall, three miles away on the east side of Somerville, and parted ways. Rich headed to Home Depot and my family to Clarks Bostonian Outlet, a shoe store. As I perused boys' sneakers, my left arm began shaking uncontrollably as though an electric current raced through it. Panicked, I combed the aisles for Mark and thrust my quivering limb toward him when I saw him.

"I can't control this," I said, coherent but freaked out.

Mark led me to a bench typically used for trying on shoes and gently held my shaking arm in his lap.

"Okay, try to relax," he said as he sat next to me, placed his arm on my shoulder, and tried to coax me toward calm.

But then I felt that familiar seizure grip on my gut, only it was huge. I couldn't control the shuddering in my arm. There was no way I could deep-breathe my way out of the symptoms. I could barely keep myself upright at that point.

And then I was out.

❧ ☙

When I came to, I lay in a hospital bed. I recalled the scene at Clarks shoe store.

Oh crap. I had a seizure-how disappointing! Can we not tell my father and Chris? Worried it might lead to a horrible outcome, they'd been wary of my decision to have surgery. I desperately wanted to hide my brain's failure from them.

Even after a friggin' brain surgery, the misfiring neurons could still take over! How could this be? If brain surgery couldn't stop them, what would? Words floating above me from a voice near the bottom of the bed interrupted my thoughts.

"This emergency surgery is in no way related to the first surgery you had in April."

Huh? Surgery? What the . . . ?

I wanted to ask questions, but I couldn't speak, as there was an endotracheal tube threaded down my throat. Later, I would learn that the better part of a day had passed since I was in Clarks. During that time, EMTs had rushed me to Massachusetts General Hospital, MGH, where Mark gave neurosurgeons permission to perform an emergency craniotomy—removing a bone flap from the skull to access the brain. The doctors removed a subdural hematoma, trigger for the stroke-like shaking and subsequent grand mal seizure I had experienced.

As I reemerged from the anesthesia-induced fog, I tried to make sense of the doctor's words, but overpowering thirst distracted me as well as irritation in my throat from the tube.

Then I saw Mark by the bed. *Oh, good. Mark can tell me what happened! But wait—I have this annoying tube shoved in my mouth. I can't talk. Ugh!*

Mark saw me stirring and took my hand. "You're up," he noted as his lips curled into a weak smile.

Wait, hadn't we done this before? I ignored the creepy déjà vu and did the only thing I could to express myself. I traced out letters on Mark's green shirt: F-U-C-K.

Mark's feeble smile spread across his face. I imagine how reassured he must have felt when he saw I could spell a word. Looking back, the hope that simple obscenity probably conjured was almost comical—except for the critical situation.

Much later, I read the email Greta sent via Lotsa Helping Hands shortly after I sketched out that expletive.

> Happy to report that Laura is talking, and her memory and thinking are completely intact! We are so relieved . . . . She will be at Mass General Hospital today and tomorrow as she recovers from this hopefully short detour.

Over the next day, I stewed in the hospital bed. *How could this happen when everything had been going so well?*

I'd been so functional while recovering. Just the other week, I volunteered to be the "mystery reader" for Liam's first grade class. Our downstairs tenants gave notice that they were moving in the fall, so I posted a Craig's List ad. A couple days before the emergency operation, I'd shown the apartment multiple times.

With a possible new fall consulting gig in mind, I perused job listings. I received Daniel's e-invitation and marked my calendar for his July 4 wedding. Yet, there I was flat out in the neurosurgery unit at MGH and so doped up on anti-epileptic drugs and painkillers that it hurt to think when I was awake. Hopefully, I'd be able to attend my brother's wedding.

That day launched our bummer of summer—far longer and more intense than the "short detour" Greta mentioned in her post. The week following the craniotomy was the worst ever. Nurses repeatedly roused me so I could verify the year and president's name. The doctor had doubled my levetiracetam and administered an opioid painkiller. I reeled from surgery's side effects.

I just wanted to sleep. Enormous pressures in my head had turned sitting in bed and talking into enormous tasks. I was a woozy mess. Mark often stayed around, reading the paper. He'd picked up the email notifications where Greta left off. Each time I woke, I noticed the same tentative smile cross his face as he saw me come to.

"You're up," he observed.

"I, uh—barely. I'm dizzy, and I just want to sleep more."

"That's okay then. Go back to sleep."

"Where are the kids now?"

"They're home. Rich stayed with them until Dan could get there. They tag teamed it."

I felt grateful as I imagined Rich and Dan coordinating the baton passing by cellphone.

"Funny that Rich was around for yet another one of my grand mal seizures."

"Yeah. He took the kids to Legoland. Their staff gave us free tickets when they saw the ambulance taking you away."

"I can't believe this happened. The seizures were supposed to stop after brain surgery, but they've gotten worse."

"The doctor said they still might stop."

"He did? Tell me more."

My head was spinning, so I couldn't fully take in Mark's explanation, but I would hear it again from the doctor and eventually read it in Mark's Lotsa Helping Hands posts.

The trigger for the grand mal at the grand mall (as Liam liked to call it) was different from the one for my pre-surgery seizures. A slow dripping of blood from a low-pressure vein stretched near the site of the first surgery between my skull and brain caused Saturday's seizure. The dripping happened during a couple weeks after the April surgery.

Pressure between my skull and brain lining created a hardened blood clot or hematoma that strained my brain. When the strain became too much, I lost control of my left arm at the shoe store. Apparently that pressure might cause anybody to have a seizure, but given my brain's wiring, I was even more likely under the circumstances. With the hematoma removed, the doctor said I was no more likely to have the decades-old, chronic problem with neuron misfiring than I was before the previous weekend.

I recalled the day I banged my head on the bottom of the freezer door while retrieving an ice cube tray. It was a hot day in May, and I really wanted a cold drink. *Maybe that impact caused the hematoma to develop.* It was impossible to know for sure—I needed a nap.

I'd had a grand mal seizure despite the temporal lobectomy—even that drastic step failed to keep my seizures under control. Had my carelessness with the ice tray caused the hematoma to develop? I stewed, my mind a morass of fear, guilt, and anger.

Surgery was supposed to stop—or at least decrease—seizures, not increase their severity. It was certainly not supposed to lead to hardened blood clots forming in my brain's lining!

Doom and gloom settled over me like a scratchy wool blanket. I felt uncomfortable in my skin. A nurse interrupted my fretting, so I gave her my name, date of birth, and Barack Obama's name, and she informed me that the attending doctor was going to speak with Mark and me.

Dr. S reviewed my records and reiterated what Mark said about the blood clot likely spurring the seizure.

"The clot is removed, and the CT scan showed a decrease in swelling," said the doctor. She examined my scalp. "The incision is clean and dry—it's healing nicely. We scheduled a follow-up to have the sutures removed."

Oh right—more staples in my head. I winced.

"We think you can go home today."

I had been grousing to Mark over the possibility of missing Daniel's wedding on Friday, but once Dr. S announced my release, I was nervous.

"Are you sure it's okay to leave?" I asked.

"Yes," Dr. S said. "We've doubled your levetiracetam, which should prevent seizure activity, and as I said, the swelling is down. But you should probably not be left alone at least for a few days, and you need lots of rest."

I took hope in Dr. S's words, which implied seizure-freedom was still a possibility. Maybe I could replace that rough wool covering with a soft silky bedspread. Of course, her initial orders of bed rest and 24/7 Laura-watch left me feeling shackled-a prisoner of my brain.

I felt so spacey that even the prospective cab ride home seemed daunting. Hopefully, my brain wouldn't go off the rails and bring on another seizure. The possibility scared me, but I was too tired to protest the plan, and part of me was happy to go home.

"You should avoid exercise other than walking for six weeks," Dr. S added. With that, she sent us home with a bottle of opioid medication and a list of forbidden activities including twisting, heavy house cleaning, and aerobics. I couldn't imagine doing anything other than lying down.

When I got home, I trudged upstairs and collapsed in my bed. Thankfully, we'd finished renovating the attic into a master bedroom complete with its own bathroom and a good air-conditioning system. I appreciated my comfy digs. I could do nothing but crank up the AC and nap. I slept on and off, my life a drug-induced blur.

I spent two days sleeping. The kids stayed with next-door neighbors when I first got home-Daniel had passed the childcare baton to them at the end of the weekend so Mark retrieved them when we got home. He kept them downstairs, so I could sleep. When I occasionally woke up, I was slammed by the ache in my head. I took a dose of opioid medication and drifted back to sleep.

Mark wanted to go to the office midweek, so Greta came by to take over Laura-watch. I didn't like being under fulltime surveillance, but I was grateful for Greta's presence. On early Wednesday evening, I woke up hungry from my drug-induced nap and sought out food and company downstairs. I found a peach in the kitchen and sat down next to Greta on the couch. She had brought her kids with her. Eliana and Gabriel were close in age to Liam, and I could hear the four cousins' banter from the bedrooms.

"Sounds like they're having fun in there," I said nodding toward the kids' rooms. "Have the cousins been getting along well?" Four kids, age range five through eight, meant a lot of young people's needs to balance. At least Greta was a teacher by profession, so she could handle it.

"Yeah, they've been fine. The girls are in Amelia's room. The boys are in Liam's.

"Mark called a little while ago," Greta added. "He's on his way home. We'll head back to Natick when he gets here."

"Good. Thanks for coming today."

I bit into the perfectly ripe peach and savored its sweetness reminiscent of long summer days and homemade pie. Then I noticed a tingling in the fingers on my left hand like the sensation brought on when circulation is cut off and your hand falls asleep. Suddenly the vague tingling progressed farther up my limb to uncontrollable stiffening in my left arm.

Oh, Crap!

"Laura! Are you okay?" Greta looked panicked as she reached for my shoulder.

"I don't think so. I'm probably going to have another seizure!" The kids heard Greta cry out and came to the living room.

"Is Mom having another seizure?" Liam asked as Greta called 911 from her cellphone.

He looked scared. I longed to scoop him into my arms and assure him everything would be okay, but I was physically incapable and totally uncertain. Instead, I listened to Greta giving data to the respondent on the other end of the call as the seizure hijacked the rest of my body.

"My sister is having a seizure," she reported, reciting our address. *Greta will make sure the kids are okay,* I thought.

My left arm still shook, flopping up and down against the velvety red couch cushions as I lay scared on my back. I knew it all headed to nowhere good.

Later, Greta told me that when she saw the left side of my face drooping and my limbs stiffening, she felt compelled to take the peach away from me because she was afraid I would choke on it. She thought the symptoms looked like a stroke.

The last thing I noticed before blanking out was the pillows' cushy support beneath the length of my body. Apparently, Mark beat the EMTs to our house and accompanied me to the hospital. Eventually Greta told me that Liam asked if he could go to the hospital instead of me. When I heard the story years later, Liam's generosity and stoicism impressed and moved me. Also, it saddened me to recall that the kids had to live through another round of Mom being rushed to ER.

I woke up the next day with a splitting headache in an MGH hospital room with Mark beside me in a frighteningly familiar scenario. "I had another seizure," I said, defeated. Once again, my brain chaos had gotten the better of me.

"Yeah—seizures went on for a while after we got here. The doctors were able to stop them with medications—no surgery this time, at least," he said with a weak smile. Months later I read my medical records and learned they'd administered a tranquilizer often used as a quick-fix anticonvulsant. They also gave me a dose of benzodiazepine, often used to dispel memories from surgical procedures and with multiple potential side effects—no wonder my head hurt so badly. So, I gathered, the medical professionals must have thought surgery *might* be necessary.

"Where are the kids?" I asked. I recalled my last moments of consciousness on the couch and the fear in Liam's eyes as he asked after me. It was the second time in less than a week that chaos in my brain upended the kids' world. It broke my heart.

"Greta took them back to her house."

"Good. Dan and Jenny's wedding is tomorrow, right?" With multiple seizures and hospital stays, I had lost track of the days.

"That's right. —Tomorrow's Friday July 4."

"I wonder if I'll be able to go."

I wanted to participate in Dan and Jenny's momentous life-changing occasion. I also pursued my eternal quest to prove that yes, I could take everything in stride and carry on.

The doctors heard me grousing over possibly missing Dan's wedding and wondering if I'd be able to leave. Maybe that influenced their next steps, which were to release me that night after adding a third medication, one specifically used to thwart seizures.

I'd been on the third medication twice before. When I was six, it made my gums swell. When they put me on it in my thirties, I gained twenty pounds. Despite the negative associations, I accepted the prescription without complaint—puffy chops and an unattractive figure were minor compared to more grand mal seizures.

Though tired and cautious, I wasn't nearly as wiped as when they sent me home post surgery on the previous Saturday. It was July 3, and Boston held its fireworks a day early due to an impending hurricane on the fourth. Mark and I decided to take the subway home instead of a cab due to increased crazy traffic patterns around MGH thanks to the fireworks.

The oldest subway system in the country, Boston's trains are jam-packed at rush hour with twisting tunnels leading to regular deceleration and screechy halts. Rush hour traffic creates its own form of hell, and Boston drivers are notoriously awful—there's a reason the word Masshole was coined here. When we left the hospital, we had to choose our poison, and we chose public transit.

Once outdoors, I noticed a heaviness in my head. A sheen of sweat lined my face and torso. I feared my body might seize again, so I took small, tentative steps and attended to every sensation. I had a piece of gauze over the sutures on the right side of my head, and my remaining curls only partially concealed the white bandage.

Sitting on the train, I caught my reflection in the window. *I must look ghoulish to the other passengers. Never mind them. You're on your way home now.*

Several Red Line train stops are named after well-known institutions. We got on at Charles Street/MGH and passed through Kendall Square/Massachusetts Institute of Technology. With our train two stops beyond MGH at Central Square, I felt tingling neuropathy in my left hand. The two grand mals I'd had since the first surgery began that way.

Oh no—not again!

I wished I were back at MGH.

"I'm afraid I might have another seizure. We need to get off at the next stop."

The stretch between Central and Harvard squares always runs slow due to a twist in the tracks. The bend inevitably brings the train to a loud halt mid tunnel for at least thirty seconds, sometimes a couple of minutes. Approaching Harvard Station, I anticipated the train's break.

I tried to keep calm as the tingles in my hand traveled up my arm. *The last two grand mals didn't kick in right away. I will likely be off this subway before this tingling turns into something out of control.*

Eventually the train chugged into Harvard Square.

"Maybe we should call 911," I said as we exited the train.

"No, the traffic is miserable because of the fireworks. Let's just take the train back to MGH. It's only three stops," Mark said. I imagined waiting for an ambulance in Harvard Square, riding as it weaved through traffic into Boston, and the ambulance bill at the other end. At the time, Mark's proposition made sense. Based on the past week's experience, if I were going to have a seizure, we had enough time to get to the hospital. I agreed to the subway plan.

Relieved to see a train approaching almost immediately, we trotted down to the inbound subway platform. The train ran without delays, so we were back at the Charles/MGH stop in ten minutes. The tingles had traveled up my left arm and onto my face. Completely coherent and terrified, I realized my brain was delicate and my body was succumbing to a seizure's bedlam.

Mark escorted me through MGH's lobby to an administrator sitting behind a desk.

"My wife's having a seizure. She needs help," he urged. The woman looked at us like we were from Mars.

"What's your name?" she asked me.

I rattled it off. I was lucid, though the tingling sensations had spread to the other side of my face. "I was discharged less than an hour ago," I added.

"Address?"

"She was just discharged a little while ago!" Mark repeated. "Can't you find her contact info in your computer?" he implored the administrator as she typed something on her keyboard.

"Oh, here we are. "So, you're still at 64 Hooker Ave?" she asked.

Were they serious? Did they really think my address had changed in the last hour?? There's no time for this now!

"That's right. All of the information is the same." Mark said. "I think she's going to need a doctor any second. Can you please get somebody?"

Even in my panicked state, I could see he was agitated. The woman continued to double-check answers on her electronic intake form. Before I lost consciousness, I saw her call over her shoulder to another staff person.

❧ ☙

I woke up a few hours later in a hospital bed, Mark beside me in a chair. I felt like I'd been walloped in the head—dizzy and still achy from the surgery, but at least I didn't have a tube shoved down my throat. I could talk, though forming words took great effort.

"I guess they shouldn't have sent me home today." My seizures had gotten the better of my brain—again. I was demeaned. I probably should have insisted they keep me inpatient, but I'd wanted to attend Daniel's wedding. Even more, I wanted to be okay.

The next day was Independence Day. I wanted to be independent and free of those damn seizures, already! "Who's got the kids?" I asked. Before the seizure hit, we'd been heading home to take them back from the neighbors, and I knew Geoff and Afsana couldn't have kept them indefinitely.

"They're with Joyce and Richard for now," Mark said. "Greta offered to take them if necessary. Hopefully, you'll get to go home soon."

I disregarded Mark's optimism. The thought of leaving the hospital intimidated me. *Who's to say I won't have another grand mal? How could I possibly recover from the craniotomy if I keep having big seizures? Was the brain surgery a failure? If I keep having grand mals, I'll say yes.* The grand mals followed by the MGH back-and-forth put me on a merry-go-round I needed to get off!

I had another grand mal the next day while Mark and my friend Laurie were visiting. Mark sat in a chair at the bedside, and Laurie stood against the wall near the foot of the bed. We recounted the past week's dismaying details when I felt the tingling in my left hand again. I don't think I had much time to tell Mark what was happening, nor did I need to. We both had plenty of experience with it.

115

I showed Mark my shaking arm as irrepressible moans escaped from my mouth. While the episode was a bummer, I appreciated the setting—in a hospital with experienced staff and surrounded by people I loved. And my kids were elsewhere.

In the end the hospital kept me four more days. Mark stayed with me at MGH on July 4, and Greta took the kids to Dan and Jenny's wedding. She wound up keeping them at her house for the rest of that hospital stay.

On Sunday, Dan and Jenny visited me at MGH and recited their wedding vows to each other. As I lay in bed sporting a hospital johnny, they sat side by side in chairs by my bedside, their faces turned toward each other.

"I promise to continue to love you more every day for the rest of our lives," Jenny said, "to grow and change with you and to embrace each new adventure and curve we encounter as well as to savor the down time.

"I will love you honestly and openly and unconditionally," she continued. "I will be your rock during difficult times, and I will keep striving to be easy with the world, to be present, and to enjoy the short time we have together on earth. For the rest of my life, you are my priority."

Dan let go of Jenny's hand, fished out a piece of paper from his pocket, and read to Jenny.

"I love you more than these words can express," he proclaimed. "I promise to always be here for you, to always stand by you and support you, to teach you and learn from you, to take care of you and be taken care of by you, to be your best friend and to love you unconditionally forever.

"Will you be my wife?"

Their heartfelt promises filled the fluorescently lit room, overpowering the drone of beeps from heart monitors and other life tracking equipment I heard in the hall. I appreciated Dan and Jenny's gesture to include me in the ceremony, despite my dizziness and over-medication haze. Mark wasn't with us, but I conjured up his image, as I listened to Dan and Jenny's vows to care for each other through thick and thin. He and I will weather this, I thought.

The July 4 seizure was the fourth I'd had in seven days, so I'd dubbed it "grand mal week." The previous time I'd had four grand mal seizures, they'd spread out over seven years. What was going on? Frequent big seizures could *not* become a "new normal" for my brain.

Thankfully, the hospital didn't discharge me too quickly. Given the week I had, I was far from being out of the woods. The hospital was the safest place for me. Meantime, they cranked up the anti-convulsants.

Bummer Summer

They released me July 8 with instructions to take a massive drug cocktail comprised of three medications, including a further increase in my levetiracetam, and I dutifully agreed. The potion would keep me perpetually dizzy but enduring that would avoid more grand mal seizures.

The doctor instructed me to take lorazepam if I felt a seizure coming on and then call my doctors. She also advised me to stay under adult supervision 24/7 for several weeks. My brain was still in a precarious place healing from the hematoma, so blood leakage might stimulate more seizure activity.

After MGH released me, Mark took on implementing a Laura-watch plan, ensuring another adult was always with me. Both my mother and father wound up staying with me a couple of afternoons. I hadn't been that reliant on a parent for decades, and it felt weird. Demeaned by dependence, I slogged through the initial days, scared I would seize.

Mark dropped the kids off at their day camp programs, and other people—friends, family members, or sitters—picked them up. A couple days later while my mother was with me, my legs suddenly buckled under me. I was heading from the couch to the kitchen when I fell. The physical disarray I felt lying on the dining room floor reminded me of a seizure, but I remained coherent. I wasn't seizing, but my body had gone out of control in a different way.

"Are you okay?" my mother asked, extending an arm to hoist me off the floor and lead me to the couch.

"Yeah—I mean kind of. I'm not having a seizure, but this is weird. I can't stand up right now. We should call the doctor."

"Do you think we should call 911?"

"No. Let's call Dr. P and have her paged. This isn't a seizure."

I was attuned to every creeping sensation in my head, wayward flutter in my belly, and tingling in my fingers, and I felt none of those. Lack of muscle coordination worried me but paled in comparison to seizures.

We got through to Dr. P, and she said that muscle coordination loss could be due to the phenytoin I took as part of the seizure-control protocol, but could also be caused by post-surgery fatigue. She advised me to continue my seizure watch-relaxation plan at home. "See, no need to go to the ER," I explained to my mother, both of us relieved.

The regular neuropathy in my fingers unnerved me. Whenever I felt the prickling, I feared another grand mal about to hit, so I often scarfed down lorazepam. Three days after my release from MGH, my father accompanied me to an appointment with my neurologist and the neurosurgeon. Although it felt strange to have my father minding me, I was grateful to have a second set of ears with me, with Mark at work.

The doctors sat across the small room, Dr. P viewing my records on the computer screen, Dr. A with a folder in her hand.

"We have some good news," Dr. A started. "Your CT Scan results show that the hematoma is getting smaller, which indicates your brain is healing." Dr. A's square glasses gave her a bookish appearance, and she presented as somebody who would give an accurate assessment. Even so, I was frustrated.

"I just had four grand mal seizures in a week! That's never happened before. Should I expect to have them on a regular basis now?"

What if every seizure I have going forward is this big? If I had seizures as often as I did prior to April, I couldn't function independently, couldn't take care of my kids. This was not supposed to be the outcome from surgery.

"No, hopefully not. The seizures you had last week were not related to the ones you had prior to your first surgery. These grand mals originated from a different place in your brain, triggered by the subdural hematoma. If we can stop the grand mals now, once the hematoma fully heals, there's a good chance you won't have them anymore."

"Well, I often felt like I might have one," I said, consulting my notes. "I felt tingling in my left hand several times since I left MGH. I assumed the neuropathy might lead to another grand mal, so I took lorazepam three times."

"You need to cut back on the lorazepam," Dr. P said. "It can be addictive, plus it stops working when your body gets used it."

"So what do I do if I feel like a seizure might be starting?" The question gushed from my mouth in an exasperated rush. The doctors' directives presented a wretched Catch-22: Don't have any more grand mals—stop the pattern before it set in. But if I took the quick fix anti-convulsant, I'd become addicted and ultimately it wouldn't work.

"We're going to give you a prescription for a liquid tranquilizer, diazepam, which is faster acting in solution form. Only take it if you're certain you're experiencing seizure symptoms. The neuropathy isn't necessarily a seizure indicator—it might be your brain's recovery process triggering the tingling. Or even medication side effects. Consider the diazepam a last resort."

I was depleted when we left, quiet in the car while my father drove us home.

"You need to take it easy," he observed. "You probably shouldn't be left alone for a while."

"That's easier said than done, you know. Mark's been coordinating Laura-watch by email, and people only have so much time. Not to mention finding people to take the kids to and from day camp."

"Hire somebody if you have to. I can help pay for it. You heard what the doctors said—it's critical that you stay seizure-free the next several weeks. Somebody needs to be with you to administer the diazepam or call 911 if another seizure hits."

Dad's no-nonsense brusque tone came from fear. I was scared too. That night, Mark posted an ad on Care.com. By the end of the weekend, Mark got the liquid diazepam prescription filled at the compounding pharmacy in a neighboring town. He vetted through the Care.com responses, and hired an older woman named Lovering to help with Laura-watch. Apparently, she had experience providing personal care in people's homes.

Lovering showed up Monday as Mark left to take the kids to camp and go to work. Stressing that she call him right away if I had any seizure activity, Mark gave her cursory instructions. Lovering hung out and read in the living room while I sat in my office or rested upstairs in bed. I resigned myself to what felt like a peculiar arrangement, just as strange as having my parents with me.

By late morning, I realized that a slight rash I'd noticed on my chest on Sunday had spread to my neck and intensified. Initial small bumps above my breasts had extended beyond my collarbone and transformed into large red splotches. I found Lovering reading in the living room.

"I think I'm having an allergic reaction to one of my anti-seizure medications," I told Lovering. "Or maybe the combination of all of them," I explained.

"Should we call 911?"

"No. I'm going to call my neurologist. I don't think this is an emergency. Not yet, anyway."

When I explained my symptoms, Dr. P instructed me to admit myself to Brigham and Women's right away. On the heels of my recent experience checking in at MGH with its unpleasant and insensitive quiz, I distrusted her directive.

"Will they be expecting me?" I asked.

"When you get to ER, tell them I told you to have them call the neurology unit. I'll tell my staff you're coming as soon as we hang up."

Lovering drove me to Brigham and Women's Hospital, and Dr. P's instructions worked. After a short wait, staff checked me into a room in their neurology unit. I sent Lovering home-after all, there were medical professionals monitoring me. I'd called Mark from the car while en route to the hospital. He'd offered to come, but there was no need. I told him to keep things going at home.

I lay in the hospital bed and adjusted to the room. Although dizzy from drug cocktails, I could still calculate data on my life circumstances. This was my fourth hospital admission in sixteen days, and the eleventh one of those days that I'd spend in a hospital. I was relieved to be at Brigham despite the crappy numbers. Mired in the depths of seizure watch, I felt terrified by every tingling sensation I experienced. The hospital was the safest place to be, and we didn't have to pay a stranger to watch me. Plus, the doctors would get me off phenytoin.

Dr. P said I needed a different third medication to ensure I stayed seizure-free. I spent four days in an over-medicated sleepy blur as she gradually added carbamazepine while tapering me off phenytoin. By the third day at Brigham, I had a new symptom—nystagmus, or uncontrollable eye blinking. *Ugh! Another body part not under my command? Really?* I was pleased that my lids were rapidly flapping up and down when Dr. P had planned a visit to my room. "See this blinking—that's out of my control," I explained. "Is that from the phenytoin?"

"It's likely related. We're taking you off the phenytoin, but it can take several days for the medication to clear out of your system. The blinking can also be a side effect of carbamazepine. Most likely, the multiple drug combination is too much. There's a reasonable chance this will go away when you're off the phenytoin."

Hopefully Dr. P's prediction was correct.

She was on the mark about the medication mixture, which was too much. I slept on and off during the day, and my head ached from pressure, as though it was waterlogged all the time. But the mega-cocktail kept the seizures at bay, and until the hematoma healed, I had no other option. I desperately wanted some tangible proof of recovery, which was elusive as I lay there in the hospital, my head swimming in drugs. Only with a positive CT scan result could I get what I needed.

On my last day—the fourth—at Brigham, I emailed Dr. A using my cellphone. I implored her to schedule my CT scan earlier.

I've spent thirteen of the last twenty days in-patient in a hospital. I'm still at BWH now as Dr. P and her colleagues attempt to concoct that perfect mega-drug cocktail to safely get me through my healing progression. In addition to the allergic reaction, the drug cocktail makes me sleepy, dizzy, and just yesterday caused uncontrollable rapid eye blinking.

I'm all in favor of doing whatever it takes to get through this vulnerable phase for the greater goal of lifelong seizure freedom— really, I'm not being a complainer. I wonder if it's possible to reschedule my July 29 CT scan a little sooner, like July 25 or July 28? Even one or two days fewer on the drug cocktail would be an improvement. Thanks for the great surgery experience in April. Wish me luck.

After I left the hospital, Dr. A emailed back the same day. She agreed to reschedule the CT scan for July 25 and meet with me after the test to discuss the results. I finally had something potentially positive to look forward to. If the CT scan showed that the hematoma was still healing, they'd be able to decrease my meds a tiny bit.

᠅ ᠅

Greta picked me up from Brigham and Women's in the early afternoon and helped me fetch the kids from their day camps. First Liam, who attended Parts and Crafts in a renovated old Somerville storefront revamped into a crafty shop space for kids. The kids spent their time in a space teeming with art supplies and power tools. They created projects, ran around the local playground, or ice skated at the nearby indoor rink.

Greta and I parked a mere block from the site, but the short walk exhausted me. When I asked for Liam, a staff member told us we'd have to wait while they found him in the playground.

As Greta and I sat on the beat-up leather couch, fatigue progressed into tingling sensations in my arm and on my face. I focused on the feel of the leather against the backs of my legs— cool and sticky against my warm skin. Then I tried to concentrate on my breathing and recalled my doctor's words. *The tingling isn't necessarily a seizure*. I focused on that thought and ignored my prickling skin. Suddenly Liam was before us, and Greta squatted on the floor to embrace him.

"Hi Liam. Mom's here to take you home today."

A flicker of joy crossed Liam's face. Then he took stock of the others in the room and stopped short. Even at the tender age of seven, he had some degree of self-consciousness when expressing affection for me in front of friends. Perhaps his reservation also

123

related to all the recent back-and-forths to hospitals. With my repeated in-patient stays, he may not have trusted that I would really stay home.

"Here. Give me a hug, too" I said, pulling him to me for a quick squeeze.

"You're coming home now?" Liam asked as he pulled away.

"Yeah. We're going to get Amelia and go home. Greta's going to visit until Dad gets home," I added, hoping it would reassure him.

"Time to go," Greta declared cheerily.

We drove across Somerville to pick up Amelia, who attended a city-managed summer camp at the kids' school. When we arrived, I immediately spotted Amelia among the kids climbing over and under the tan playground structure in the woodchip-covered schoolyard. At least we wouldn't have to wait for somebody to find her. Liam saw Amelia running across the planks of the slack bridge and ran toward her, calling as he did.

"Mom's here!"

When Amelia heard Liam, she stopped chasing her friend and scanned the yard, her glance landing on Greta and me. She scrambled down to the ground and streaked past the structure toward us, throwing her arms around my legs in a hug.

"Mommy—you're back!"

"Yes, I am. Today's the last day of camp. Dad's on vacation next week," I added.

"Yay!" Amelia gushed. *Yes, yay.*

Once Mark got home that night, we wouldn't need to make Laura-watch arrangements for ten days. I couldn't wait simply to *be* with my family for a stretch. Hopefully I could also avoid seizures. Greta and I found staff, signed Amelia out, and drove home, where I collapsed on the couch.

I was spent. The hot heavy air filled our unairconditioned second-floor unit and stifled me.

"I need to turn on the AC upstairs and rest," I told Greta.

"Good idea," she said.

"Mark should be home by 6:30. I bet we can find something on television for the kids to watch. Then we can visit in my room and listen for them."

"Perfect."

Greta found something on PBS and joined me upstairs. "They're hunkered down in front of *Cat in The Hat*," she informed me. "*Curious George* is on after that."

"Good."

Mark would arrive home shortly after the shows ended, I calculated. I wanted to take advantage of the quiet window and chat with Greta, but as soon as I got into bed, sleep's grip dragged me down. "I'm sorry—I need to sleep," I said.

"That's okay—sleep is great for you right now."

I settled in bed and fiddled with the AC control as Greta perched at the bottom of Mark's side.

"I can't believe I'm this tired. All I've done today is lie in a hospital bed and pick up the kids," I said.

"You've had a few rough weeks. Give yourself a break. Sleep—you need it."

"Thanks."

With that, I drifted off.

By the time I woke up, Greta had long gone, and Mark was home from work. I lay in bed taking solace in the comforting sounds of Mark and the kids putzing around downstairs. I heard the clanking of silverware against plates. I longed to join them for dinner.

When I opted for brain surgery, I chose the more invasive, supposedly more effective procedure. Since late April, every seizure I'd had was bigger and scarier than the pre-surgery seizures. And now I couldn't be left alone. It wasn't what I signed up for.

I was swindled as if I'd ordered a toaster on eBay listed as "good condition" but, when it arrived, sparks flew out of the wall socket as I plugged it in. My tweaked brain felt like that used toaster, neurons flying everywhere. Given my dependent and drugged-out condition, my brain surgeries seemed as helpful as a hazardous toaster.

The doctors claimed it was temporary. Once the hematoma healed, I'd be far less seizure-prone, and they could reduce the meds. My woozy days equaled a thick, yucky pond I had to swim across. On the far end of the water, I glimpsed a beachy shoreline and, just beyond that, a warm inlet where I could dip and rinse. That lovely bay was seizure-freedom and pre-surgery drug levels. Plagued with questions, I had to slog through the mucky bog.

What if the doctors were wrong? What if Laura-watch and overpowering medication cocktails were part of my permanent landscape?

I roused myself out of bed and joined my family downstairs.

❧ ❧

Summer ticked by in a slow-motion, drug-induced fog that left me perpetually dizzy. A combination of the hematoma's after-effects and the anti-epileptic drugs, AEDs, continued to cause regular tingling sensations in my hands and face. That side effect played a mean joke as it mimicked seizure precursors I'd had during disastrous grand-mal week. Initially, I panicked every time the tingling started. Sometimes it lasted a few minutes, sometimes an hour or more. When the prickles began, I recalled the grandest grand mal in the shoe store and fell into hyper alert. *Is this going to progress into a seizure? Am I about to shake uncontrollably?*

On July 25, Mark and I met with Dr. A after my CT scan. She reported that the hematoma had further decreased in size. "Your brain is definitely healing," she told us.

Relief washed over me.

"We still need that third medication to keep you safe."

My pride bubble thanks to three seizure-free weeks burst. I was too fatigued to truly live my life when I took three medications.

"But you're on the right track," she added.

"Didn't you say we could lower the carbamazepine if the results were good?" I asked.

"We can titrate it down, but we have to do it slowly so the seizures don't start again."

Take heart—a slow decrease is better than no decrease.

"What about Laura-watch?" Mark asked. Between friends, family, and Mark's vacation days, we'd managed 24/7 coverage without hiring somebody since my release from Brigham eleven days earlier. While it was nice to have friends' company, requesting their help felt like an imposition, and arranging coverage created its own job, which Mark did. "I need to go back to work on Monday," he added.

"Once Laura's been seizure-free for thirty days, she can go unsupervised," Dr. A said.

I'd been given another milestone to achieve. The craniotomy had reduced my goals to the ability to plod around my own house alone—a depressingly low bar. But clearly, Laura-watch remained part of the yucky swamp I had to cross that summer. I visualized the relaxing shoreline at the other side and continued to make may way across.

Thirty days from July 4 was August 3, nine days away with two weekends in between, so we required only five more days of Laura-watch and I knew my friend Jackie would cover one. Assuming no seizures, I'd be independent again after that. I was agitated by the summer's morass of calculations and alarming sensations, but I buoyed my spirits imagining that lovely warm inlet—seizure-freedom and independence. I took it day by day, noting each one that went by seizure-free as inching toward the beach.

As summer progressed, I learned that not every prickle had to lead to a seizure. In fact, none of them did. I created a ritual. Every time I felt the creeping sensations in my fingers, I rhythmically tapped my thumbs against the pads of my other four fingers, while silently repeating my new mantra: "I'm taking so many AED's, I can't possibly seize!" It calmed me somewhat, but the finger tingles still made me edgy that summer. In September, the neuropathy serendipitously occurred during an EEG, which showed no seizure activity. After that. I was undaunted by the finger prickles.

In mid August, Dr. P agreed to start the medication reduction plan. She insisted on keeping the third band-aid drug carbamazepine. But my three-thousand-milligram levetiracetam dose was twice what it was prior to the April surgery, so she agreed to taper it slowly. The taper took eight months before I was back to my original levetiracetam dose. In the meantime, I lived with the side effects: dizziness, lethargy, and extreme thirst.

August unrolled and seizure watch morphed into sanity watch, my effort to stay grounded in the face of fear and extreme restlessness. I didn't really want to go out on hot humid days in my overly drugged state, so I arranged for adult visitors whenever possible. My brother Daniel came by one day. I felt well enough that

I poked around my kitchen, excitedly preparing a pot of black bean chili with spinach, one of the easiest entrees ever. Unfortunately, we didn't have any scallions in the house—the critical condiment that makes the dish yummy. I texted Dan, who came bearing my requested purchase from the local artisan market.

"Here you go," he said, handing me the small bunch. "They charge per scallion there—a quarter each, so I only got four."

"Perfect. Thank you!"

I was delighted I could cook, and that the meal would be as delicious as ever thanks to Daniel. I added wilted spinach leaves to the simmering pan and brought the pot to a boil before turning the flame down low.

"Let's go to my air-conditioned bedroom," I said. "This is basically done, and I'm ready for a break." We retired upstairs, me spread out on the bed, Daniel on a chair nearby, and chatted about nothing consequential.

"Do you use those much?" Dan asked, nodding at the elliptical and stationary bicycle tucked in the corner of my room.

"Well, not now—no strenuous exercise until after August 28. But when I'm not recovering from brain surgery, I do. Usually four times a week. Now, I'm lucky if I can putter around the kitchen without collapsing," I said with a small smile. "These days I spend a lot of time up here in bed. But, hey, I wrote this song while lying around. It's called *So Many AEDs* —short for anti-epileptic drugs," I explained. "Ready?"

Daniel nodded, and I belted the words from bed. I tapped my mattress to create a backbeat in the style of an eighties hip hop tune (think *The Message* by Grandmaster Flash and the Furious Five), and gently bobbed my head:

> I'm taking so many AEDs, I just can't possibly seize.
> I'm taking so many AEDs, I just can't possibly seize.
> They got those neurons under control.
> My persnickety brain they needed to cajole
> 'cause no seizures is the ultimate goal.
> I'm taking so many AEDs, I just can't possibly seize.
> I'm taking so many AEDs, I just can't possibly seize.

Kudos to the docs who got me through this month with
no grand mals,
but the AED cocktails—they got their flaws.
Say "Screw those orders because
they must OD you on drugs to win seizure wars."
I'm taking so many AEDs, I just can't possibly seize.
I'm taking so many AEDs, I just can't possibly seize.
To cease to seize is key-
to the life that's meant for me!

"That's it," I said looking up from my chicken-scratched journal. "It doesn't scan perfectly. —It's still in rough draft form."

"That's okay. It's clever—I get the point."

"Good. I've been lying around here so long, I needed to do something constructive—like making a point."

In recent years, epilepsy practitioners and advocates began referring to anti-epileptic drugs as anti-seizure medications, or ASMs, rendering my comfort phrase and rap poem outdated. The language shifted because the term AED is perceived to have negative connotations toward those with epilepsy. Also, while the drugs may effectively keep seizures at bay, they don't necessarily put the kibosh on an epilepsy diagnosis. So, the phrase ASM is more accurate. But in 2014, AED was still the accepted nomenclature.

≈≈ ≈≈

A couple weeks later while the kids were in day camp, I took my first walk alone to Davis Square just under a mile from our house. I'd gone more than the requisite thirty days seizure-free, so given Dr. A's directive, I felt fairly confident I wouldn't have a seizure. The meds still caused thirst and fatigue, so I grabbed my full water bottle. Summer sun beat down as I walked the narrow familiar streets, heavy hot air providing no relief. By the time I got to Davis, I'd downed the full quart of water, and I needed more.

I could have purchased a quart of seltzer from any number of places in the square, but my primary care doctor's office was right there on Elm Street. The staff was kind, and the office equipped with a free water cooler. Given that my desperation for water due to a medication regimen ordered by a doctor, albeit a different one, it seemed appropriate to take advantage of my doctor's free cooler. When I walked in, I vaguely recognized the admin assistant behind the glass pane that separated her from the office. Hopefully, she'd recognize me, too.

"Can I help you?" she asked, her voice lilting up, her face friendly.

"Can I fill my water bottle here?" I asked. "I'm a patient of Dr. D. I just walked into the square, and I'm super thirsty from all the post-surgery meds I'm on. I need some more water." *I've been Dr. D.'s patient since 1988. She'd want me to have the water.* Despite my insistent thoughts, I felt vulnerable standing on the other side of the glass pane. I'd just guzzled a quart of water, and walking a mile left me desperately thirsty. *Will my body ever go back to normal?*

"Sure, help yourself," the assistant replied.

"Thanks." I filled the bottle, slurped down half of it, and then filled it again for the walk home. The medication cocktail was key to seizure freedom. Yet the meds caused inordinate thirst that left me parched, craving water with the same intensity that I yearned for seizure-freedom. To this day, I stash a full water bottle in my bag when I go out, as it's only a matter of time before I need some. I take far less medication now and the thirst is not as intense as it was that summer—a small nuisance compared to having seizures.

I ran my errand—possibly a simple staple from CVS like dental floss or maybe a prescription refill. I retraced my steps home and made it back hydrated enough and seizure-free with one simple errand successfully completed unaccompanied. As I entered the apartment, my sense of achievement mitigated the post-excursion physical exhaustion.

Yippee! I made it home alone!

The Healing Journey Continues

By late August, I decided I was well enough to take a short trip to Providence, Rhode Island, with Mark and the kids. I wasn't feeling a hundred percent—it would be almost a year before I came close to that—but I was stir-crazy from spending the summer in bed, so we took the trip anyway. My levetiracetam dose was lower, and the lacosamide dosage back to its level prior to the emergency surgery, but the third drug, carbamazepine, guaranteed regular long bouts of dizziness. My doctors insisted I needed it to keep me safe.

"Your brain is still delicate while it heals from surgery. A seizure could reverse the healing process," Dr. A said. "Also, the longer you go without a seizure, the less likely you'll have another one. Your brain is still unlearning the seizure response. The third med is critical to ensuring that your brain quits its automatic seizure response pattern."

The meds made me feel crappy. but experience had taught me Dr. A was right. Seizures beget seizures. I couldn't afford to have one. There was nothing to do except suck it up and live with the side effects. But I wasn't going to let them stop me from taking the trip.

We stayed at a hotel and planned several kid friendly destinations—Block Island, the children's museum, the WaterFire festival. Sometimes I hung back in our room and napped while Mark took the kids out, but often I plowed through the fatigue and tried to enjoy the change of scene. The first day, I relaxed on the beach and watched Mark and the kids at the ocean's edge. The sea breeze cooled off my sweaty neck, exposed to the sun with my hair pulled back. I slurped water from my omnipresent purple water bottle. I dozed off, woke up, and noted with relief that I felt mostly okay.

I relaxed in the hotel the next morning while Mark and the kids went swimming and then opted to join them on the trip to the children's museum. I expended my energy in careful spurts, tagging after Mark and the kids while they explored life-sized mazes and experiential water toys. When exhaustion slowed me down, I used a bench as my vantage point. Mark sat next to me and placed his arm on the bench's back behind my shoulders. "How're you feeling?"

"Okay." Mark caught my tentative tone.

"You sure?"

"Kind of tired, actually," I admitted as I slugged the last of my water. "And I need more water."

Mark heard the urgency in my voice.

"Here. I'll get it for you."

I was grateful for Mark's attentiveness as he ambled to the restrooms, found the water fountain, and returned the full bottle to me. Feeling near giddy with relief as I rehydrated, I sucked the water back.

"Thanks—that's better. I think I have enough momentum to move on." But by the time we went out for lunch, my mini energy reserve had gone. *Geez, all I did was walk around the children's museum! Damn this slow recovery and medication side effects!* My limited oomph exasperated me.

Lunch included Amelia's tantrum over the food as she dug in her five-year-old heels over the restaurant choice, and by the time we returned to the hotel, I was fatigued. I lay low for a few hours while Mark and the kids went swimming.

By evening, my energy level had gone up, so we strolled down to the Waterplace Park to see the Providence WaterFire lighting installation. With the Woonasquatucket and Providence rivers winding along its downtown streets, Providence reminded me of a mini-Venice.

That night the rivers were ablaze with miniature bonfires, lit at sunset for the WaterFire festival. Sidewalks overlooking the water were lined with wood-slatted fences to keep pedestrians from falling into the river. The railing was also ideal for leaning against, I thought—the walk to the river had sapped my post-dinner second wind—but it was lined with people. At last I spotted an unoccupied stretch of fencing.

"Let's stop here," I directed. We arranged ourselves at the fence while I searched for my water bottle, chugged a few sips, and took in the view. Dozens of people paddled kayaks on the river between the blazing braziers. The kayakers all had an illuminated Japanese koi fish affixed on a stick mounted in their boats. When I squinted, I saw patches of bright colors above the water—magenta, purple, lime green–they reminded me of my childhood light up toy with the psychedelic-colored plastic pins that fit into a black pegboard. The cheery distraction helped me enjoy the evening.

My reprieve from discomfort ended the next day. I woke up desperately thirsty and gasping for breath.

I guzzled some water and lay quietly in bed, as everybody else was still asleep. I inhaled slow, deep mouthfuls of air to steady my breathing and my nerves.

Damn this breath shortness!

Where all three of my meds listed breath shortness as a side effect, I attributed the symptom mostly to the drug cocktail. But when I'd mentioned that to my neurologist a few weeks earlier, she insisted it couldn't be the meds. Though seizure-free, I felt like I lived in the body of a frail eighty-year-old.

I'd hoped to work part-time in the fall, but that morning, I needed to reassess my plans—both for the autumn and for the day. The previous day's agenda had overwhelmed me. I sent Mark and the kids off to the pool followed by further explorations of Providence and kept myself on bed rest.

"Are you sure you'll be okay?" Mark asked.

"I'll be fine. You're going to the pool in the same building. When you go exploring, stay nearby, and keep your phone handy. I'll call your cell if I feel anything weird. I'm probably just going to sleep. Remember, I'm taking so many AEDs, I can't possibly seize."

My family left, and I spent the day drifting between naps and a half awake woozy state, panting and attempting to quell my unquenchable thirst.

❧ ❧

Later that week, I had an appointment with my neurologist. I reiterated my theory about the breath shortness, that the symptom kicked in when they added a third medication. All three medications list breath shortness as a side effect, and the combination made it hard for me to breathe, according to my hypothesis. Dr. P agreed the symptom was troubling and ordered an electrocardiogram. I was skeptical, but I followed her advice. It didn't surprise me when the test came back normal.

About two weeks after our trip to Providence the doctor *finally* agreed in mid September to begin a slow tapering off carbamazepine. Although *she* wasn't sure that the meds caused my breathing troubles, Dr. P was convinced that my brain was stable enough to remain seizure-free without the third medication. She sent me home with a slow taper plan that spanned eleven weeks.

Breathing complications persisted for the first month, leading to scheduling an October echocardiogram and pulmonary function tests. When they both came back normal, Dr. P suggested I try an epinephrine inhaler to rule out asthma. My father had asthma, but how likely was it that I'd developed it at age forty-seven? Again dubious, I dutifully sucked on the inhaler on two different days when I intermittently struggled to breathe for several hours. I felt vindicated and relieved when the inhaler had no effect. I *knew* I didn't have asthma.

In addition to assessing my heart and lung functions, my neurologist and neurosurgeon required a battery of neurological tests throughout early autumn to monitor my brain. That season, my life was comprised of regular trips to multiple hospitals for a series of alphabet soup testing: EKG, ECG, MRI, EEG, CT scan. Thankfully, Amelia could attend public pre-kindergarten in September, so I made the appointments while the kids were in school.

Once I decreased the carbamazepine by thirty-three percent, breath shortness abated slightly. It would totally go when I completely weaned from the medication. All those diagnostic tests and inhaler experimentation ended up a waste of time. I decided to drop Dr. P around the same time I cut back the carbamazepine.

❧ ❧

In the meantime, Dr. A, the neurosurgeon who performed the first elective brain surgery, gave me an appointment in response to an email I'd written on the heels of our Providence trip. I brought my question list, although I knew Dr. A probably wouldn't have clear answers to them. Dr. A's fallible sagacity was apparent from the email I received from her assistant in response to my biggest concern: How much longer would I feel like crap? Shannon's note said Dr. A couldn't put a time frame on it, as every case is unique.

I recalled a conversation I'd had with Dr. A after the elective brain surgery in April. She'd said that, while my brain healed, new tissue would grow in, filling the empty space from the piece she'd removed during the temporal lobectomy and that my healing brain resembled that of an elderly person. Four months later, as I recovered from the June emergency craniotomy slice and dice, my brain looked like a centenarian's according to Dr. A's example. Yet, I felt certain medication side effects caused some of my woozy fatigue.

I would never know for certain how much of my fatigue was due to medication and how much was due to brain recovery.

I read news articles on my cellphone to distract myself from the frustrating conclusion. My appointment fell on primary election day, so I skimmed stories about polling results for the Democratic gubernatorial contest as I waited for Dr. A in the sterile hospital office. I rooted for Donald Berwick, one of the underdog candidates. I (correctly) suspected he didn't stand a chance, but his progressive platforms inspired me enough to follow the news and cheer him on.

I looked up from my phone when Dr. A walked in. She shook my hand and sat down at the desk.

"It's primary day in Massachusetts. If you're a Massachusetts resident, don't forget to vote," I announced—my small effort to increase voter participation. It surprised me when my words brought tears to Dr. A's eyes—Dr. A wasn't the type to cry. With her angular features, bookish glasses, and toothy smile, Dr. A reminded me of my former stepmother. Mary was emotionally detached by nature, so I found Dr. A's tears bizarre. I'd never seen Mary come close to crying. On a visceral level, I knew the emotional display made Dr. A uncomfortable, too.

In awkward silence, I witnessed Dr. A's distress while ticking off in my head possible reasons why she might be crying. Maybe the primary election was a sore spot between her and her partner. Perhaps they'd had a spat over breakfast that very morning, and my comment riled her? Or maybe she had scary unexpected test results.

That's it —she's about to break the news that I have a brain tumor, and she can't bear it.

But then she relayed the positive MRI results which showed no evidence of permanent damage from the hematoma. My brain was on a healing trajectory. Despite the good news, Dr. A wept. I wanted to comfort her—an automatic maternal response—but recognized it as situationally inappropriate. If anybody deserved comforting, it was me. I decided to ignore Dr. A's tears.

"So, if my brain is healing, how much longer before the ongoing fatigue goes away?" I asked. Just as her assistant said in the email, Dr. A couldn't give me a clear answer.

"If you feel worn out, you probably need to take it easier," she reiterated. Her tears shook me so much that her vague unsatisfying advice didn't annoy me. I suspected the reason she wept had nothing to do with primary contests or imagined tumors. Dr. A just felt relieved to see me well enough to pay attention to the bigger world around me.

❧ ❧

In late October, I met Dr. E, my new neurologist. I really wanted to like her better than I liked Dr. P. In addition to my annoyance at Dr. P's insisting on unnecessary tests, I'd sought Dr. E out because I found Dr. P a bit cool.

Brigham and Women's Hospital refers their brain surgery patients to social workers in case they need help navigating the recovery road. When I met with Keith, the social worker assigned to me, he nodded sympathetically when I explained my grievances during our appointment.

"We need to find you a doctor who's also a mensch," he proclaimed. In Yiddish, that word translates to a person of integrity. In English, the word has evolved to mean a good-hearted, dependable solid person. I wanted Dr. E to fit both definitions.

By the time we met, Dr. E had all the alphabet soup test results. She had straight brown hair, blue eyes, and a warm smile. After Dr.

P's cool manner, the latter was important—it almost made up for my discomfort over the fact that she was five to ten years younger than me. (I'd become an ageist over time, equating youth and inexperience.) She shook my hand warmly before sitting down in front of the computer with records of my brain surgery and test results.

"It's very nice to meet you," she said, briefly scanning the computer screen. I was grateful when she turned her eyes to meet mine. Hopefully, she'd taken the time to read through everything before we sat down.

"You've been through a lot," she noted. "How are you feeling now?" *Glad she asked.* I reached into my bag and pulled the folder which contained a myriad of my own records. Dr. E was going to get a comprehensive answer. I presented my chart documenting every side effect I'd felt each day since my August appointment with Dr. P and all the drug level test results I'd taken since summer 2013. One by one, I calmly lobbed my bullet point list of questions at her.

"How likely is it that the seizures will stay away?" I asked. There was no guarantee. Dr. E gave the standard answer. Seventy percent of surgery patients remained seizure-free.

"But I didn't stay seizure-free. It seems like I'm among the thirty percent who have seizures after surgery."

"Not exactly. The post-surgery seizures were brought on by the subdural hematoma. They were a different type of seizure."

"Yeah—they were much worse," I chimed in.

"Right, of course. But my point is they were different. You still haven't had any complex partial seizures since the first surgery in April, right?"

I conceded it was true. "And last week's MRI results look great. Your brain is healing. There's a seventy percent chance you'll remain seizure-free."

At least the second surgery and hematoma hadn't decreased the percentage. "Okay, seventy percent. I'll take that. But can we get the chronic dizziness to go away? I was dizzy for over an hour more than half the days since my last appointment. I'm still taking almost twenty percent more levetiracetam than prior to the surgeries, and my levels are far higher than they used to be. Do you think we can lower it again?"

Dr. E wasn't sure to what extent brain healing caused the dizziness versus medication side effects.

"You need to move slowly, Laura. We're already tapering you off the carbamazepine. You don't want to have any more seizures. We need to hold steady on the levetiracetam for now. Once you're off the carbamazepine, if your brain is stable, we can try to get the levetiracetam down to where it was last summer."

Dr. E was right. I didn't want to have any seizures. I had to accept her plan. At least my shortness of breath had significantly diminished thanks to the carbamazepine taper.

"Okay, no levetiracetam adjustment," I agreed. "One more question. Since all the drug package inserts list breath shortness as a symptom, and my breathing troubles started right when the neurologists began this mega-drug cocktail regimen, *why* do you think the doctors insisted that they couldn't be related?"

"Because you're the first patient they met with this symptom."

Her answer annoyed me. If the package inserts listed breath shortness as a side effect, how could I be the first? *There must have at least been a lab rat that came before me. What a waste of time and money spent on diagnostic tests and inhalers!* Dr. E had nothing to do with it of course, so it wouldn't be fair to rage at her.

I gave her my best suggestion. "You should write an article about my experience and get it published in the *Journal of the American Medical Association*. Then other patients won't have to go through this next time."

I tossed a few more questions at Dr. E, and she patiently answered. To the best of my knowledge, Dr. E didn't write that article. But she took my acerbic nature in stride during that difficult period. She's always warm and clear, so she's still my neurologist.

By November, I was still on three meds but close to the end of the carbamazepine taper. While I experienced some dizziness every day, days when I felt fatigued for more than an hour rarely occurred. Wooziness came in predictable waves that correlated with my medication regimen, so during the day, I prophylactically drank lots of coffee to mitigate it. Fatigue levels would only decrease as I tapered the carbamazepine—it was just a matter of time.

I still tracked every racing, prickling sensation that crept across my hands and face and each flutter in my tummy, as I didn't know for certain whether to identify them as simple pre-seizure symptoms or medication side effects. To this day I don't know for sure. The small physical stirs paled in comparison to my pre-surgery, complex partial seizures—just a gentle odd tingle on my mouth or cheek. But they reminded me of my seizure precursors, so they unnerved me.

❧ ❧

While walking to Davis Square to run errands, I noticed a weird prickling on my lips. *Is this going to morph into the uncontrollable lip smacking brought on by a complex partial seizure?* I took stock of my surroundings: I was on Highland Avenue, the late afternoon summer sun descending over the brick structures. I saw familiar storefronts—the martial arts studio where Liam had previously taken classes, the Blue Shirt Café that sells overly healthy wraps.

I snuck a sidelong glance at the kids. Amelia was content riding in the stroller and Liam, walking by my side. They were oblivious to the tingling in my mouth.

I took stock of my body. The weird mouth sensation decreased, and I remained completely aware of my surroundings. I silently counseled myself. *Breath deep, keep your cool. You're fine. These odd symptoms have never progressed into a seizure.*

The symptoms subsided, and I continued walking. I remained cognizant, albeit slightly rattled.

❧ ❧

When I reached out to Dr. E about such bouts, I took heart in the content and expediency of her response. Even if what I experienced were pre-seizure auras, she still considered me seizure-free. Given that the surgeons had cut out the bad part of my brain, she thought I was unlikely to have a bigger seizure.

Buoyed by Dr. E's assessment and the drop in side effects and symptoms, I focused on reestablishing my life footing. I joined the kids' school improvement council as a volunteer parent representative. I submitted applications for part-time grant writing jobs. I coordinated childcare for multiple doctors' appointments and occasional date nights away from kids.

I still had seemingly random setback days when I experienced multiple troubling symptoms—extended fatigue, a long bout of neuropathy in my hand, or a couple of suspicious tummy flutters. I comforted myself with Dr. E's recent words–she still considered me seizure-free—but days with symptoms frustrated me.

I took to redirecting my aggravated energy to health assessment and research and meticulously analyzed trends in my symptoms. I compared the trends with changes to my medication regimen. I searched online for subdural hematoma and craniotomy, which led me to academic sites quoting medical studies and self-care sites like Healthline.com. Fascinated by the details, I read the articles. One reads:

> An acute subdural hematoma can only be treated in an operating room. A surgical procedure called a craniotomy may be used to remove a large subdural hematoma. In this procedure, your surgeon removes part of your skull to access the hematoma. Then they use suction and irrigation to remove it.

I imagined scalpels cutting into my skull—an image painful to the point of the surreal. Reflexively I brought my hand to the right side of my head, where two inches of thick curls had grown over my scars. I combed my fingers through the short hair and felt for the scars. I could visualize them because I examined them during my weekly deep-conditioning treatment.

The emergency craniotomy scar was higher than the elective surgery scar. The less invasive elective surgery incision left a low rainbow curve over my right ear. The craniotomy scar is a U-shaped arc that runs over the first welt. Although the arch is narrower, the bumpy scar line is twice as wide as the lower curve. That procedure was an emergency response done in haste. The neurosurgeon had to use staples to seal the incision, and they remained in my head for eighteen days. Removal of those staples was one of my most painful surgery-related experiences.

Yep—that rutted hair-free scar line proved I'd survived the gruesome procedure I'd just read about! Reading the straightforward depiction reaffirmed what I experienced. No wonder I still felt like crap. Greedily taking in information, I clicked from link to link:

A subdural hematoma is a collection of blood outside the brain. The bleeding and increased pressure on the brain from a subdural hematoma can be life-threatening.

One article quoted a sixty-five percent mortality rate for patients my age recovering from a subdural hematoma. Another imprecise study rated mortality in the range from fifty to ninety percent. Reading those statistics slammed home the enormity of my second surgery. I kept a higher number—eighty percent mortality rate—in my head, as it felt more empowering. But even lower survival odds and written account of the procedure emboldened me. A doctor had cut into my head twice and lobbed out chunks of my brain. The second time, they'd used who knows what tools to suction and drain out a blood clot. If I could endure that, there wasn't much I couldn't recover from.

Luckily, I had somewhat recuperated when I read all that, and at that point, there was no doubt I was a survivor.

I recalled my September appointment with Dr. A. No wonder she broke out in tears. Dr. A was thankful to see me alive on primary day. Did the hematoma develop due to over-stretching a vein during the first surgery or from the impact sustained when I bumped my head on the freezer door in May? I'll never know, and the answer is irrelevant.

Looking out my window, I saw it cold enough that puddles from the previous day's rainstorm had frozen into a thin layer of black ice, tricky for walking. Navigating the precarious sidewalk might serve as a metaphor for the perpetual skate on thin ice of my pre-surgery life. Back then, having a seizure was an eventuality, akin to losing my footing on a frozen pond. But I couldn't predict when or why I'd fall, who would witness it, or where it would happen. I'd unexpectedly landed on my ass and hauled myself up countless times for decades.

Leading up to elective brain surgery when I told family and friends about my decision to have the temporal lobectomy, many people commented on the brave choice I'd made. While that's correct, it's also true that living with uncontrollable seizures required far more courage than both brain surgeries combined. Hell, I had no choice about the emergency craniotomy—that was Mark's decision.

My doctors had told me it's possible for neurosurgery patients like me to go seizure-free for years and then inexplicably start having seizures again. The ice beneath me is thicker, but it will never be a hundred percent solid. Despite inherent lack of guarantee, I felt thrilled and empowered to have that thin brittle frozen pond replaced by a dense, smooth skating rink.

Gratitude welled inside as I read the alarming medical details. I was thankful that the day my brain imploded, I was near a good hospital that had the staff and resources to treat me successfully. I was especially grateful to the neurosurgeons on call that day.

My emergency occurred on June 28, 2014, the first Saturday of summer. I imagine those doctors probably out enjoying the sun with family or friends when MGH paged them. Had it not been for their specific skills, I could have easily died that day. Every June 28, I send a silent thank you their way and check their online profiles to see what they've accomplished.

The surgery details also increased my appreciation for life and my undependable seizure-freedom. Every month, week, even day that I didn't have a seizure, I could celebrate my brain's newfound homeostasis.

Surviving the hematoma also decreased my tolerance for difficult conversations that go nowhere. Whenever I sense that I'm figuratively banging my head against the wall—meaning I can't change the other person's mind because their life-lens is permanent—I recall the scars on my head, and the craniotomy description, and I stop the conversation. Even figurative head banging is a bad idea for somebody with my life experience.

Every person has a birthday, and everybody's life eventually comes to an end, but only a small subset of us has a near-death anniversary. Mine is the day I would have died were it not for the skills of the MGH neurosurgical staff and my body's will and strength.

I am thankful for all of it.

The Last One

I was still seizure-free about a year later and thrilled that ongoing seizure-freedom might be a real possibility. The emergency craniotomy was seventeen months behind me. While I sometimes experienced a small tingling in my face that may have been neurologically triggered, I'd had no seizures for almost a year and a half.

I continued to monitor all my symptoms for Dr. E, and my dizzy-spell tracker chart looked good. I looked forward to the upcoming winter solstice and lengthening of days. Longer term, I was counting down to June, as that's when Dr. A said it would be safe for me to consider driving. I live in a city with decent public transit, so I'd handily managed my whole life without a license. But I loved the idea of one, especially the additional independence it would provide. I wouldn't have to rely on others to run errands efficiently, get places, or take my kids to their extracurriculars.

One Friday night, we cleaned up after dinner, and looked forward to a low-key evening together and the weekend ahead. As I left the kitchen and walked toward the couch, I heard a loud popping noise like firecrackers going off. Mark was near me, also walking to the living room. I looked at him, and I could tell he hadn't heard anything. Then I heard the popping noise a second time—a loud and distinctive rattling. Also undisturbed by the noise, the kids continued playing in Amelia's room.

"Did you hear that loud crackling noise?" I demanded. As I asked, I felt something amiss in my core—I remained standing, but I was off balance like I might swerve and fall over at any moment.

"No, I didn't," Mark replied. I determined that the noise was in my head and related to the topsy-turvy sensations in my body. I followed Mark to the living room, sat down next to him on the red couch, and wrapped my arms around him like a little girl. I moaned uncontrollably.

By then, we all realized I was in the throes of a seizure—a big one. The bizarre auditory hallucination so rattled me that I wasn't scared. But as seizure's jagged clutch overtook my gut, I clung to Mark for comfort. I'd been seizure-free more than a year, but here we were again. I was in the grip of a seizure, but aware of my surroundings.

"Liam, call 911," Mark commanded. Liam grabbed the phone from its cradle and paced across the room as he dialed.

"My mother's having a grand mal seizure," he said into the phone. He was silent a moment, then ticked off our address. Liam was only a month shy of his ninth birthday—I was struck by his composure and courage. Mark and I had talked with him about how to call 911 two years earlier. I'd felt guilty and glum about possibly saddling him with that responsibility. At the time, he'd shrieked "No," but that night, he executed the call perfectly. I heard sirens in the distance as despondency set in. I was exasperated that Liam and Amelia had to witness another round of the ambulance coming for Mom.

I was still conscious when the medics arrived. They lifted me from the couch and lugged me down our winding front staircase to the ambulance waiting outside. Mark had called on neighbors to keep an eye on the kids, so he sat next to me as I lay on the gurney in the ambulance. I vaguely noted some beeps inside the vehicle emitted by equipment I couldn't see, and I registered the siren as the EMT tore down the Somerville streets toward MGH.

❧ ☙

Woozy as hell, I came to in a hospital bed. I saw Mark dozing in a chair and longed to call to him, but when I attempted to raise myself onto my elbows so I could project my voice, my head reeled. I gave it up. There were no tubes in my mouth, so I probably hadn't undergone any surgery, I concluded, but the pain in my mouth rivaled the soreness in my head. My tongue was lacerated because I'd bitten it, a common physical response during grand mal seizures.

144

"Mark," I called to him a couple of times before I could rouse him. He wore Dad clothes—jeans and a gray sweatshirt with Westie the Wolf, the kids' school logo. He came to, caught my eye, and smiled.

"Is it Saturday?" I asked.

"Yes." Mark checked his watch. "It's 1:00 p.m.," he said. I did the calculations.

"I've been asleep almost twenty hours?"

"You had several seizures in a row last night," Mark explained. "They had to give you sedatives plus extra levetiracetam to stop them." That explained the reeling dizziness. And my poor tongue—I probably gnawed it multiple times.

"Where are the kids?"

"I got Rowan to take over from Geoff and Afsana. I wasn't sure if you'd be awake yet." Rowan was our most recent sitter.

"Good." I didn't want to rely on our neighbors for too long. They'd been called in before, and they had their own young child.

"I'm sure the kids will want to see you soon, though," Mark said.

Yes, of course they would. But after the experience of 2014 grand mal week, I wasn't ready to go home.

"Maybe you can bring them by this evening after I nap—or even tomorrow. I want to be sure I don't have another seizure."

"Sounds good to me," Mark said with a wan smile. His disheveled hair and droopy eyelids proved he'd slept in a chair the previous night.

"You should go home," I said.

"Are you sure?"

"Yes. This was just a seizure—no surgeries. I'm doped up dizzy, but I'll sleep it off. The kids want to see you, too. Plus, you can bring them back for a visit."

Though I was disappointed by the setback and I felt like crap, I wasn't too worried. "This is by far the safest place for me to be," I reminded Mark. "Besides, I know why I had that seizure."

"Because you just had the week from hell?" Mark referenced work deadlines and a sudden in-person meeting with Liam's guidance counselor about Liam's acting out.

"That didn't help, but I had that seizure because I brought the lacosamide down to zero last week. Looks like my brain needs it to stay stable."

A few minutes later, the neurologist on call came by. I learned that in addition to dosing me with sedatives, they gave me 4,000 milligrams of levetiracetam and added back the lacosamide at 100 milligrams twice daily. "I usually take 1,250 milligrams of levetiracetam a day. No wonder I'm so tired," I noted.

"That was an emergency measure to stop the seizures," the doctor explained. "We only gave you a thousand milligrams this morning." He had dark hair, dark stubble and brown eyes, and was probably in his thirties. "The good news is the CT scan showed no new hemorrhaging or lesions on your brain. Also, the subdural hematoma that developed last year has continued to clear."

While that was good news, it didn't stop the reeling in my head.

"Can you lower the levetiracetam?" I asked.

"I think we should leave it at a thousand milligrams twice daily for now."

"That's a lot for me," I said.

"You need to work with your neurologist," the doctor said. "Given the seizures you had last night, I have to leave the levetiracetam where it is."

Case closed. The next few weeks would be hard as I readjusted to the medication changes. By chance, I already had an appointment with Dr. E a few days later. *She'll help me figure this out.*

I suspected the seizure was probably just a setback. I went to the bathroom and examined my tongue in the mirror. White cauliflower-like bumps outlined the gash where I'd chewed on it. I felt immense pain, and I'd inflicted it on myself! My brain's strong misfiring neurons bowled over my pain receptors' response. It would be two weeks before I could eat anything besides applesauce without strategizing about where to put the food morsels in my mouth.

In addition to my wounded tongue, I'd burst a blood vessel in my left eye. The white had a bright red line going through it that looked more worrisome than it felt. At least it didn't hurt. Despite feeling high as a kite from anticonvulsants and sedatives, I could function.

I called my boss, explained what happened, and told her I needed to take Monday off. Mark dropped by later with the kids and the library book I'd instructed him to bring. I was watching TV in bed when they arrived. My tongue hurt, and I felt dizzy from the meds, but I was cognizant.

"Mommy!" Amelia shouted, running toward my bedside. "You're up." Liam approached the opposite side of the hospital bed, so I was flanked by both of them with Mark hovering in the doorway. I put an arm around each child.

"Mom, what happened to your eye? Are you okay? Are you coming home today?" Liam's concern and Amelia's jubilance pushed me past my aches and pains.

"I am okay. My eye doesn't hurt. But I'm not coming home yet."

"Aww. Why not?" Amelia asked.

"I want to be extra sure. They sent me home too soon the last time, and I had more seizures. I don't want to put us through something like that again," I said.

"Okay," she agreed. They stayed while I ate the breakfast they'd brought, and then I was ready for a nap.

"We're going to go to the zipline on the Esplanade," Amelia announced.

"Good. Thanks for bringing me the fried egg sandwich. It was much better than hospital food. Have fun on the zipline. I'll come home soon."

I stayed at MGH two more nights. I slept, rested, and read the novel Mark brought me. I probably could have gone home Sunday night, but given my 2014 experience, I felt MGH owed me the extra sense of care and security. By Monday morning, I'd finished my novel, and I was ready to leave.

❧ ❧

Two days later, a pending sense of doom hanging over me, I entered Dr. E's office. I feared she wouldn't let me taper my levetiracetam dosage back to 1,250 milligrams and also that she would extend my two-year post-surgery milestone and tell me I wouldn't be eligible to drive the following summer. I sat anxiously next to her desk as she reviewed MGH discharge records on her computer. When she shifted her gaze from the screen to me, I made my case.

"They had to add the lacosamide back all at once, and they brought the levetiracetam up more than fifty percent, so I feel awful," I said.

"Yes, 2,000 milligrams of levetiracetam is definitely too much for you," she agreed. "With the addition of lacosamide, we can bring the levetiracetam down to 1,250 milligrams daily."

I breathed a sigh of relief. *Whoopee!*

"We've got to do it slowly."

Yes, of course. Everything about seizure recovery was slow—I knew that.

"You can lower it by fifty milligrams every two weeks."

"That sounds good. Can I still consider getting my driver's license this summer?"

"As long as you remain seizure-free for six months, you're allowed to drive," she replied. I did the calculation: Six months from December 4 brought me to June 4. *Woo-hoo—I'm going to get this!*

I broke into a smile. "That's great."

Dr. E told me to return in six weeks so she could monitor the levetiracetam taper. It took three months to bring the levetiracetam back to my baseline level.

During December, most days I experienced severe dizziness for multiple hours. I tracked it daily on the spreadsheet I'd created in 2014. I shared my spreadsheets with my neurologist at every appointment. Dr. E usually gave them a cursory glance, compelling me to point out relevant patterns or incidents I'd noticed. During my initial post-surgery years, if I were woozy for more than thirty minutes, I highlighted the chart boxes yellow. The "dizziness/light-headedness" column for December 2015 was mostly yellow. As I expected, the month was a total bust.

I was working part-time writing grants for a nonprofit called GirlsLEAP. On workdays, I had an hourlong Red Line commute to Dorchester, kids to take care of when I got home, babysitting schedules to coordinate. Some evenings, I had to attend school improvement council meetings or kids' activities. As any working parent knows, balancing that full plate poses a juggling act that requires skill, systems, and oomph. I had the first two requirements down, but the extra levetiracetam hampered my energy levels. I hated that unexpected miserable déjà vu as if I were living through a scaled down version of my post-surgery summer. But if could get through 2014, I'd get through this, too.

Prior to December 4, I'd gone exactly seventeen months with no seizures. I could trace the latest seizure to a decrease in lacosamide dosage. The seizures I had in 2014 were related to the subdural hematoma. Despite such clear connections, my seizure patterns frustrated me. All the significant seizure activity I'd had since the first surgery were grand mal seizures that landed me in the ER. While regularly having complex partial seizures was a nuisance, those didn't require trips to the hospital and major medication adjustments that fatigued me for weeks.

Brain surgery was supposed to put an end to those challenges, but in some ways the ordeals had grown bigger. My agitation prompted me to email Dr. A. I explained the situation and asked her why all my post-surgery seizures had been so different. In addition to being less frequent and much more severe, they had different precursors. Why were my seizures so much worse post-surgery? Wasn't surgery supposed to help? I ended an email to her with a plea for advice:

> When I'd gone almost a year and a half seizure-free, I was optimistic. Dr. E says there's still reason to be optimistic now—that since I did so well on two meds for so long, there's a good chance I can go back to being seizure-free again. But this all feels extremely unfair, and as you know, epilepsy sucks. There's no need for me to recite the string of expletives that goes through my head when I think about all I've been through—you get the idea. I'm reaching out now, as I thought perhaps, you'd have useful insights for me.

I hadn't seen Dr. A in well more than a year. As I hit send, it occurred to me that she may have closed my case and feel no obligation to respond. *But the last time we met she'd been moved to tears.*

Dr. A emailed the next morning. She said it wasn't unusual for seizure precursors to change—that difference confirmed that the brain areas that previously caused my seizures were successfully removed. Dr. A referenced the pre-surgical tests they'd run, showing brain abnormalities.

"This means that there is the potential for other areas to generate seizures," she wrote. Again, this is not unusual," she continued.

> It is quite expected that the seizures might be different since they are originating from a different part of your brain and that they might be more severe since in one case there was the subdural and in the other a medication had just been discontinued. Your brain has a predisposition to have seizures, something which, again, is common in patients with medically refractory epilepsy even when surgery is successful. So, I suggest you stay optimistic and connect closely with Dr. E to get you back on the best possible track to control your seizures. Warm regards.

Although Dr. A's reference to everlasting seizure susceptibility of my brain was sobering, I loved her detailed logical explanation. Her words provided me hope that seizure-freedom was still achievable, encouragement I desperately needed.

December 2015 was the last time I had a significant seizure. It was also the last contact with Dr. A. Almost as much as I loved the comprehensive content of Dr. A's email, was that I could count on her to write me back.

Beyond Recovered:
Life Through the Lens of an
Invisible Disability

License Liberation

In spring 2016, I was counting the days until the requisite six months passed after the previous grand mal. I wanted my learner's permit so I could learn to drive.

I spoke with my father on the phone as June approached. "I'm going to start taking driving lessons next month," I said, my voice bursting with pride and excitement.

"Are you sure that's a good idea?" he asked. "I mean, what if you have another seizure?"

"I had that last one because I stopped taking lacosamide. Otherwise, I've been seizure-free for almost two years since the brain surgeries. The doctor said it was okay," I added to make him feel better.

"Well, I wouldn't do it if I was in your shoes."

Damn. Dad could be a Denny Downer! His response disregarded my colossal personal triumph—I'd gone nearly seizure-free for two years. *Stop raining on my parade, Denny*! Although I was vexed, I knew his reaction came from genuine fear and concern, so I chose my words carefully.

"If you had undergone two brain surgeries, you might feel differently. After everything I've been through, I'm not passing on this opportunity."

"Okay." I was pleasantly surprised when Dad let the topic drop after that. While I found the exchange agitating, I knew Dad's pessimism was indicative of his perpetual tendency to see the glass as half empty. Getting my driver's license was icing on my seizure-freedom cake. After the journey I'd completed, I was going to have my cake and eat it, too—with every bit of frosting I could get! Half empty glasses be damned—the frosting is my favorite part.

Carving out time between professional commitments and fitting in lessons when the kids were in school, I worked with three different driving instructors through the summer and autumn.

Driving lessons cost fifty dollars an hour, so I also needed to practice on my own. Occasionally, I imposed upon friends. Despite his concern, my father even accompanied me a couple times, although he lived in Maine. But after instructors, I practiced with Mark more than anybody else. The kids weren't old enough to be left alone, so I'd often practice while running local errands on the weekends, Mark at my side, the kids in the backseat. Those flawed learning conditions were perfect for intermarital spats.

Mark is a meticulous polite driver who boasts about having never received a ticket for a moving violation. When I mentioned that to one of my driving instructors, James Bruno replied, "He's just never been caught. Everybody makes mistakes." Rather than putting the pedal to the metal, Mark slows down when the traffic light turns yellow. I have total confidence in his driving abilities, but practicing with Mark proved challenging as he insisted on providing long critical narratives on my techniques *while* I was driving.

For example, I'd approach a rotary, which required all my acumen and concentration to navigate as I focused on signage and safely integrated myself into the traffic flow.

"You want to yield and use your signal," Mark might say, "but you don't want to stop—that just clogs everything up." *Okay, put the blinker on. The other cars have right of way. Weave in carefully.* "Also, it's considered good etiquette to stay on the outside of the rotary," he said, listing reasons why as I traversed the rotary. *How could I observe good etiquette while he was talking to me as I drove?*

"Could you stop with the long explanations while I'm driving?" I snapped at him. "That's distracting." Suffice it to say we dedicated some couples counseling time to working through issues that came up during practice. The experience was so stressful that when we go places together, I typically let Mark drive. Driving with Mark in the passenger seat brings me back to those harrowing practice sessions, which I'm happy to avoid thinking about.

❧ ❧

Massachusetts is one of few states that requires prospective drivers to bring a sponsor to the driving test. The first time I took it, I went with Mr. Bruno and took the test in his car. I followed his suggestion and scheduled the test in the nearby suburb of Wilmington. When we got to the Wilmington office for the registry of motor vehicles, I saw a teenager with somebody who looked like his mother, and I was jealous. I immediately wished I'd brought a friend or family member. I knew Mr. Bruno wouldn't provide the cheerleading I needed that day.

As soon as I slid behind the driver's wheel, I also regretted my choice to use Mr. Bruno's car. Although I'd practiced in his white station wagon, it was larger and less familiar than our sedan. Already nervous about the test, I felt my anxiety amplified tenfold by those erroneous decisions.

The examiner, who had reddish hair cropped short and a matching mustache, directed me to drive Wilmington's unfamiliar side streets. "Make a left turn when it's safe to do so," he instructed as we approached an intersection. *Wait—was it safe?*

His sharp angular features matched his curt daunting directions. They put me over the edge. When I got to the corner, I slowly turned left, but I was too wide.

I underwent the remainder of the test with the mistake hanging over my head as the examiner continued with his gruff intimidating directives. "When it's safe to do so—"

I wasn't surprised when the examiner told me I failed the test. "You were driving so unsafely, you should have paid me," he said, handing me the failure paper.

I felt sick with disappointment.

"You're not a bad driver. You just did a couple things wrong. Practice, practice, practice," Mr. Bruno said impassively.

A few days later, when a staff member at the school asked me how the test went and I owned up to my failure she said, "Think if it like the PSATs. Now you know what to expect next time."

LeeAnne was correct. Based on that first experience, I brought somebody I loved with me the next time and scheduled the test for the DMV in neighboring Cambridge, where I knew the streets. But that did not immediately translate into success. When I told my favorite driving teacher Dominique that I'd scheduled the test in Cambridge, he warned me that the examiner there was extra tough.

He couldn't be worse than that militant snark in Wilmington, could he? It turned out that Carlos wasn't meaner, but as Dominique said, he was a harsh critic. Parallel parking was my sticking point—getting it right while under observation proved to be my true challenge.

Ultimately, learning how to keep calm while under the examiner's surveillance was the key to passing my driving test. Leading up to the test I passed, I meditated every morning for a month. I had to find a sponsor other than Mark, who gave driving critiques en route to the DMV.

In the end, my buddy Rich accompanied me. We left the house early, and I practiced parallel parking beforehand on snowy North Cambridge streets.

Carlos met us out front and hopped into my Nissan. By then I was familiar with the nearby streets—and with Carlos from previous tests. I followed Carlos's instructions as I cautiously traveled the neighborhood. I knew Carlos would test my parallel parking skills last. When he did, I employed all the tricks I'd learned from my instructors and the web surfing I'd done—angling my car and lining up the view in my rearview just so.

We drove back to the DMV, and all three of us got out of the car.

"Did I pass?" I asked.

"Yes."

"Yay!"

Rich and I both cheered. When Carlos walked away, I embraced Rich in a bear hug.

"Thanks for coming with me today," I said. "Honestly, I thought my parallel parking job was no better than the last time when he said I was too close to the parked car."

"Based on his age, I bet he's ready to retire soon—maybe he decided it was okay to go easier on you this time."

"Maybe."

Was that an unintended insult? I didn't care—I was fifty years old, I had my first driver's license ever, and I was thrilled.

Getting my license was liberating—I could hop in the car to run simple errands and drive the kids to their after-school activities by myself. Adjusting to the feel of driving a car was tough, as it was worlds apart from my decades of experience with city biking. Initially, cars about to turn onto the road from perpendicular streets alarmed me. As a biker, a driver's careless turn could be fatal, so I always double checked them, making eye contact, making certain they saw me. Eventually I realized that when I was ensconced in three-thousand pounds of metal, those turning drivers were unlikely to plow into me.

My new self-perception as a car driver versus a bike rider required a bigger adjustment than overcoming my seizure-related apprehensions about driving. For years, my getting a license was both illegal and dangerous. As a driver, I am now as entitled to be on that road as any other licensed driver. Embracing that status change—and the privilege that came with it—took conscious effort.

When I see a driver waiting to turn as I'm cruising along a major road, I might try to catch their eye. If they're nosing onto the street, sometimes I even talk out loud, especially when there's traffic behind me. "You're going to wait. I've got the right of way," I say.

I know the driver can't hear me. If the kids are in the car, they scoff at my antics, but I don't care. The statement is my verbal form of the doctor's signed form—self-affirmation that I belong there.

After relying on public transit for years, it's easy to keep calm when I'm stuck in traffic jams. I allay my frustration by imagining the commute if I were doing it car-free. Inevitably, I'd be waiting for a train or bus and doing some amount of walking, all of which would take longer than waiting out the additional light-change cycles due to the cars in front of me. Then I take a deep breath and wait for the light to turn green.

The liberation provided by my driver's license came with another careful risk-benefit analysis. My seizure freedom is not guaranteed. I am obviously one of the thirty percent of brain surgery patients who *did* have seizures post surgery, although that was due to a major glitch, not a surgical procedure that failed to provide seizure-freedom. Seizures beget seizures, so the longer you go without having them, the less likely you are to have one.

My last grand mal seizure was in 2015. Since then, I've only had what I call neuroblips. They are fleeting twinges in my stomach often followed by a racing feeling in my head or a swelling sensation in my lips. The blips remind me of simple and complex partial seizures I had pre-surgery, but they're far less consequential. I don't lose awareness, and they're invisible to an observer. The number of neuroblips has also decreased over time. During my initial post-surgery year, I experienced them on thirty-six percent of days. The last time I met with Dr. E, that number was down to four percent.

My neuroblips have never progressed into a full-blown seizure, so I stopped worrying about them a few years ago. Prior to surgery, when I felt seizure precursors, I could *sometimes* keep the full seizures at bay using deep breathing and positive thinking. I use the same techniques with neuroblips, and I've had a hundred percent success rate since surgery. The blips have taken place under a variety of circumstances—at the office, alone with the kids, while on a job interview—and since they're so small, I'm the only one aware of them.

I've also experienced them on the road. The first time, I was driving on a local state highway to a friend's house. Cruising at about thirty miles per hour, I followed the curve of the road when I noticed tingling in my lips and the flutter in my belly.

Oh, a blip. They always pass, this one will too, I thought. And it did.

Another time, I felt one as I merged onto Interstate 93 near my house. I generally avoid that highway, as it's known to incite panic, frustration, and anger in many drivers. I noticed a fleeting sensation in my lips as I maneuvered the car into the right lane. *Focus on the road—the blip will pass,* I coached myself. By the time I reached a steady speed, it was over.

Whenever I experience neuroblips, I recall Dr. A's email sent after I had the last grand mal. When I noted how different that seizure was, she said the dissimilarity confirmed that the part of my brain that previously caused complex partial seizures was removed precisely.

Those misfiring neurons are like rowdy, unsupervised teens at a bash with alcohol, their drunken partying analogous to the chaos of a seizure taking over my brain. When I have neuroblips, I imagine neurons bumping against the tiny spot in my brain that abuts the section Dr. A excised with her scalpel. That miniscule mark is the parent or local official called in to stop the unruly festivities.

"Party's over," says the parent as a neuroblip sets off a small sensation I assume is a minor misfiring neuron, although I'm not a hundred percent certain. I imagine her with figurative admonishing crossed arms, blocking the neurons' trajectory. Since surgery, that trick works every time.

The pre-surgery Wada test confirmed my tendencies to depend on my brain's left side for much of my functioning, and that enabled me to have the surgery. Given that I've had grand mals out of the blue after fifteen years, there's nevertheless a chance I could have another one. When I made the choice to get my license, I intentionally relied on my left brain even more as I analyzed the odds of having a seizure while driving.

My clear, promising calculations drowned out the natural hesitations my emotional, secondary right brain offered when I envisioned a seizure on the road. The doctors say there's a thirty percent chance I might have another seizure. The percentage of time I drive is in the single digits, so when I calculate the odds that I will have another grand mal, chances are over ninety-nine percent that I *won't* be driving.

Mostly I drive near home, where traffic lights and jams abound, so it involves lots of annoying and comforting stop-starts. If a grand mal were to hit in that circumstance, I might have enough of a warning to pull over and press the button that activates my vehicle's hazard lights. Somerville streets are busy. Based on traffic flow, and my experiences with passersby, I suspect it wouldn't be long before somebody would see something amiss and call 911.

I wouldn't accept a job that required I drive the Interstate alone every day, but an occasional quick jaunt is okay. There's no question that, if I had a grand mal on the highway, it could be fatal, so I minimize the time I drive there—typically a half hour twice a month. Ironically, I'm often driving to or from my father's house then.

My Own Statler and Waldorf

In early 2017, I looked for work between consulting gigs. By then, it had been more than a year since the last grand mal, and complex seizure activity had ceased, although I still experienced the neuroblips. Those annoying flutters and distracting sensations have never progressed to a full-blown seizure.

About twice a year, the tummy flutter increased in intensity to the level of an uncomfortable nudge in my gut. It rattled me more than tingling sensations in my face, as it reminded me of the total loss of control that comes with complex seizures.

There's never a good time for approaching that edge, but in winter 2017, it occurred smack in the middle of a job interview, so it was especially inconvenient. I was being interviewed by five people, including the executive director, program manager, and human resources administrator at a small nonprofit focused on tenants' rights advocacy. I was especially drawn to Sonia, the human resources administrator, partly because she had set up the interview by telephone. She also was effervescent and made direct eye contact when she smiled. Her dark brown hair streaked with burgundy highlights, she got to ask the easy questions, like whether I preferred working in the mornings or evenings.

"Oh, I'm definitely a morning person," I said truthfully.

"Laura, your resumé says you've got extensive experience with strategic fundraising plan development for nonprofits," the finance officer tossed out.

Suddenly I felt that disconcerting internal jolt in my belly.

"Can you tell us some more about this?" the finance officer asked.

Whoa! Now that definitely felt like seizure activity—the way they used to happen. Hmm. I guess I won't get this job if I have a full-blown seizure during the interview.

I felt as though I was in the balcony seats of a theater watching the job interview on a stage below. I was Statler and Waldorf, the cantankerous *Muppet Show* characters who consistently jeer the program's cast. Only instead of taunting, I provided critical internal coaching.

Wait—take a deep breath. Try to answer the question. You've had dozens of tummy flutters, and they've never led to complex seizure activity since the surgery. You probably won't have one now either. Now answer the question. No wait—take another deep breath first. Concentrate.

I made eye contact with the executive director, focused on her blond highlights, collected my thoughts, and managed to give the group a cohesive answer about nonprofit fundraising sustainability models and how I would apply them to their organization. I took longer, deeper breaths than usual, but I don't think anybody in the room noticed. In the meantime, the lurching sensation in my stomach had subsided.

See, you're going to be fine. Totally fine.

The rest of the interview was uneventful.

When I left the building, I rifled through my purse in search of the lorazepam I keep there for just such occasions. My neurologist advised me to take that anti-anxiety medication on days I felt seizure symptoms. I hadn't had seizure activity that big in more than a year, so the pills were old, but they were better than nothing.

I downed two and walked Boston's South End streets, giddy with relief. I'd made it through the interview unscathed—nothing oddly noticeable, no major flub-ups as I answered the questions. I was thrilled.

I checked the date on the lorazepam bottle when I got home. The pills had indeed expired four months earlier. Ah, well—old lorazepam was better than no lorazepam. I made a fresh pot of coffee to mitigate the drug's effects and to celebrate.

I sipped coffee, savored a lemon chocolate chip scone, and applauded my inner coach. Years ago, I had named her Nora —she was my own Statler and Waldorf. Her name was a hybrid of my name, and the word "neuro," at the root of neurological, neurology, neurons, etc. all common vocabulary for anybody with epilepsy.

In my thirties, I'd attempted to control my seizures using a neuro-behavioral approach, without success. I journaled regularly and practiced deep breathing daily for years. The theory was that with enough practice, during the moments a seizure was coming on, I could invoke a relaxation response strong enough to calm down the misfiring neurons, before they unleashed the cascading chaos that was a seizure. Unfortunately, the technique had a relatively small impact on the number and severity of my seizures, so I ultimately gave it up. The turmoil in my brain was simply too substantial to control until I had a piece of it surgically removed. When I feel those tummy flutters now, I am confident that if I relax and breathe, the sensations will pass without incident. This has worked every time since 2014, so Nora's recent track record is excellent.

Two months after that interview, the South End-based nonprofit offered me the job, but by then I didn't want it. I already had a small contract job, and summer was about to begin, so the childcare bills would eat up most of the income. I told them to reach out to me in the fall if they were still in need of a contract grant writer. I was happy to refuse the work and enjoy a slower paced summer with the kids. But the heart of my delight at the job offer was confirmation that Nora is a great coach.

It's Not Brain Surgery

It's not brain surgery. The expression means, "It's not that complicated." As with making a perfect flaky pie crust from scratch, there's some nuance to it. With pie crust, you chill the water with ice cubes before blending it with a flour-butter mixture. It takes a bit of extra work to combine the water with ice cubes, but it's not rocket science. Since I've had two brain surgeries, the analogy about brain surgery hits me differently, especially since I know that brain surgery *is* complicated.

In summer of 2019, at the doctor's advice, we decided Liam should have his adenoids removed. After years of managing excessive congestion whenever he got colds, we took him to an ear, nose, and throat specialist, an ENT. She examined inside his nose by guiding a spaghetti-string tube attached to a camera into the depths of his nostrils.

"He has excessive adenoidal tissue. He's young enough that the tissue might go away by itself, but it may not," she told us.

After another year of wretched colds with lots of teasing at school about perpetual snot rockets, we again weighed pros and cons of adenoidectomy.

"You don't have to do this surgery—there's no guarantee it will work. The doctor said the odds of success are sixty percent. But your colds might be a whole lot easier," I explained to Liam.

"What's going to happen?"

"It's not brain surgery," I said.

Given Liam's closeup view of my yearlong healing journey, he knew what I meant. "You only go to the hospital for a few hours. They put you to sleep with medication, and then they scrape the extra tissue off the top of the inside of your nose and near your throat."

"Does it hurt?"

"You'll sleep through the operation, but after you wake up, you'll be uncomfortable for about five days, she said. Then, hopefully, your future colds won't be as bad. Think about whether you want to do it."

Liam had had enough bad colds that by the time we had the conversation, he opted for surgery. We scheduled the procedure for July 31, and I took the day off from work. Like my brain surgery, the operation entailed an early arrival with lots of waiting. I checked Liam in, only to be directed to a different floor where the surgery would take place, and we waited. Liam was subdued, reading to himself. I shared texts I'd received from my mother and Greta, wishing him well.

"Thanks," he said, looking up nonchalant and stoic from the book. But I knew he was nervous.

"You're going to be fine today—this will be over before you know it," I added.

Eventually, a heavyset red-headed nurse called Liam's name. She led us to a room with multiple beds filled with kids getting prepped for procedures.

"I'm Elinore," the nurse said. "We're going to get you ready for surgery now. Here's a johnny, which ties in the back. You're going to change into that. You can keep your underwear on. Then I'll get you ready to meet the anesthesiologist."

I helped Liam tie the confusing johnny ties. Elinore returned, affirmed that his vitals were fine, and introduced us to the anesthesiologist, who wheeled Liam in his bed to the pre-operating room. Probably in his thirties, the anesthesiologist had his hair covered with a blue shower cap. He made a big unsuccessful attempt to engage Liam with light banter, and I was relieved when he got down to the brass tacks.

"Okay," he said. "We're going to administer the anesthesia and get you to sleep. You'll breathe into a mask for a few minutes, then you'll drift off. When you wake up, the operation will be over. Any questions?"

Liam shook his head no.

"Are you ready?"

"Yes."

I stood behind the bed, my fingers stroking his bare shoulder under the johnny until he drifted off. Then they wheeled him away to the operating room and directed me to a waiting area on a different floor.

It was my turn to wait. I looked at my laptop and attempted to get some work done, but I was too distracted to concentrate. About an hour and a half later, the doctor gave me an update. "He had no bad reactions to the anesthesia, and we removed a lot of adenoidal tissue. I'm optimistic this will have a big impact on his future colds," she said.

"Is he up yet?" I wanted to see for myself that he was okay.

"Not yet. Wait here—they'll come for you when he's up."

Ugh, more waiting. I texted the update to my family and read news until another nurse called me. She introduced herself as Izaura, and I figured she was Latina. "The name confuses people— it's spelled the same as your name," she explained.

"Oh, so it's pronounced ee-zow-ra," I said, recalling my basic Spanish.

"That's right," she smiled and led me to the recovery room, where I saw Liam, asleep, splayed on a bed. He looked so vulnerable, I had to restrain myself to keep from scooping him into my arms. Instead, I found that bare spot under his johnny and gently stroked his shoulder, watching his face closely as he stirred. I saw his eyelids flutter, though they remained closed, and he made a soft guttural noise in his throat.

"Hey, it's over," I said encouragingly. "How are you doing? Does it hurt?"

"I'm okay. If you can make it through two brain surgeries, I can get through this," he said.

"Is that true?" Izaura asked me.

"Yes—five years ago during summer of 2014."

"Wow." Izaura went about her business, removing the EKG tabs stuck on Liam's chest.

"You know, they call that anesthetic the truth serum," Izaura said. "People come forward with all kinds of stuff when they come out of surgery still under its effects. They usually don't remember a thing they say."

I smiled to myself. Liam wouldn't recall saying those words, but even during those post-operative drugged-out first moments, he knew that an adenoidectomy is not brain surgery. I was proud of his foggy observation and his courage, unexpected silver linings from my own surgery experience.

❧ ❧

About a month before Liam's surgery, I experienced a suppressed appetite and barfing and I assumed I'd developed a stomach bug. But after a few days, while walking, I noticed a slight pain in my abdomen, and I was concerned. I left work early, and in the privacy of the PCP's examining room, I explained my symptoms to the nurse practitioner as she poked and prodded my abdomen.

"I think you might have appendicitis. You should have a CT scan done at Mount Auburn as soon as possible."

Two days later I was at Mount Auburn for a contrast dye CT scan. The test reminded me of the Wada test I'd had prior to brain surgery, when they injected dye through my veins. This time, I only had to ingest the contrast dye instead of having it infused through a needle into my groin. While preparation for the CT scan was uncomfortable, the appendicitis test was a breeze by comparison.

When the technician was done, she led me to a small, stark hospital room to wait. "I'm going to give these reports to the doctors to read. They should be down here in a while to share the results. I'll find your husband so he can wait with you."

She bustled away, and Mark joined me shortly after, sitting on a soft gray hospital chair next to the bed. "How did the scan go?" he asked.

"It was fine. A little like that Wada test, but less intense." When Dr. J finally entered the room forty-five minutes later, I was antsy for news. He was heavyset and balding with a trim beard and mustache. He introduced himself and thankfully got right down to business.

"The scan shows your appendix is ruptured. The good news is your body contained the pus leakage to a small site around your appendix. The bad news is that the area is extremely inflamed, and we have to check you in to treat the infection."

"Do I need an appendectomy?"

"You do, but not now. Your abdominal lining is too irritated to operate on. I'm going to put you on antibiotics to treat the infection. We can schedule the operation in a couple months after the area is fully healed."

As Dr. J left the room, a nurse appeared and wrapped a stick-on identification bracelet around my wrist to check me in to Mount Auburn Hospital. Different hospital, different diagnosis, but the bracelet instantly took me back five years to the emergency craniotomy at MGH. Just as in 2014, it was the first full weekend of summer. But this time, I was fully aware of my circumstances and surroundings.

Mark left the room to find me a breakfast snack. By the time he returned, the nurse had hooked my right arm up to an IV tube attached to a transparent sack of liquid.

"What's that for?" Mark asked.

"They're bombarding the infection with these antibiotics," I said, pointing at the bag above us.

"The setup reminds me of your brain surgeries," Mark said, his voice solemn.

"Yeah, me, too. But this will be different," I asserted.

I sent him home to take care of the kids.

"You can all visit me after the soccer game," I told him. "Bring me something good to eat and a book to read. There's a decent chance they'll release me by tomorrow."

When I met with Dr. J the next day, he had good news. "Tests indicate that your white cell count is going down," he said, "so the antibiotics are working. Given how few symptoms you had this week, your body did an amazing job containing the infection. Had you been alive during Neanderthal times, you would have been the cave woman who survived illnesses without drugs or doctors," he added.

"What about the appendectomy?"

"We still want to wait eight weeks to give your digestive system time to fully recover from the rupture and inflammation. I'm going to give you a two-week prescription for amoxicillin—take that daily."

Dr. J scheduled the appendectomy for late September. Between the June hospital stay and the operation, I had two quick follow-up appointments with him when he made sure I was okay and kept me on his roster for the appendectomy. He promised he would only operate on one patient at a time, an unsolicited rejoinder to recent press about doctors performing simultaneous surgeries on multiple patients. By the time September rolled around, I was more than ready for the procedure.

I did the pre-check-in registration by telephone as I walked home from Davis Square on a hot Friday. A nurse went over the basics of what would happen. I would be given an anesthetic before the operation. Dr. J would perform the surgery with a laparoscope—thus, no knife, as he made two small incisions with a camera to help him locate and remove my appendix. Someone would have to pick me up from the hospital.

I answered the nurse's questions and took in the information as traffic rolled past me on Holland Street. *This was nothing compared to brain surgery. I'll be fine,* I thought.

On surgery day, I took myself with a book to read to the hospital via public transportation. A nurse administered a pre-operative exam, and then there was a long wait in the fluorescently lit hospital room. I napped and read to bide the time. Dr. J appeared an hour after the scheduled 10:30 start time, and I was relieved to see him, and impatient to get the operation over with. I reminded myself that he didn't do double operations, and that was a good thing.

"Looks like you're ready for the procedure," he said.

"Yes, definitely."

Dr. J gave my abdomen some cursory pokes and prods.

"Okay, the nurse is going to administer the anesthetic and take you into the operating room."

The nurse hooked me up to an IV, and I fell asleep shortly after that. I woke up post-operation sans-appendix and with some light bruises near the incisions on my pelvis and my abdomen. They were slightly sore to the touch but nothing major. I felt a bit woozy from anesthesia—and hungry.

The procedure was a cakewalk compared to an emergency craniotomy. When Dr. J came to check on me, he confirmed what I suspected. The operation had gone well, with no complications.

I held Dr. J's description of me as the intrepid warrior cavewoman close during the weeks before and following the appendectomy. His words reinforced the self-image I'd developed post-craniotomy. Once I recovered from that invasive procedure, I felt dauntless—like nothing could beat my body. I know it sounds almost haughty, and I realize that as I age, natural wear and tear takes a toll on me. But my fifties represent the first time I've been totally seizure-free, so I am relishing my healthiest decade to date.

Since my brain surgeries, in addition to appendicitis, I've been diagnosed with epicondylitis, aka tennis elbow, and plantar fasciitis. My writer's mind notices the conditions' matching suffix *itis*, meaning inflammation, a testament to their simplicity compared to epilepsy. Epicondylitis and plantar fasciitis are significantly easier to explain to others than a seizure disorder. Brains are far more complex than limbs, appendixes, or even feet. Most important, outward symptoms of such conditions don't bungle control over my body nor scare people the way seizures do. Nobody is going to call 911 if I'm experiencing arm pain due to tennis elbow.

I've been seizure-free for more than seven years, so I am confident that my medical ordeal was worth it. Had I been warned about the obstacles, I might have hedged if my neurosurgeon had told me in advance, "Yes, seizure-freedom is attainable, but you're going to have to go through two brain surgeries and overcome some death-defying complications, which I promise you'll survive." No practitioner in her right mind would ever utter those words. But having tasted seizure-freedom, I know that, had I been provided with that information in advance, I would have made the same choice.

As harrowing as my journey was, it was less trying than navigating life while managing seizures and others' judgments of me, a statement about the challenges of living with an outwardly obvious—perhaps somewhat baffling—medical condition in our society.

If I borrow my father's lens of glass half empty and focus on the possible unpredictability of my seizure-freedom, it is more unsettling to imagine others' reactions to the seizures I might have than having the seizures themselves. I know what it's like to have seizures and live with them. While it's a bummer, I'd adjust to loss of my driver's license and to the bodily uncertainty.

I *don't* know who might be with me or where I might be if I have a seizure again nor how it would land on those around me. If I were with my family, I imagine Liam and Amelia might feel traumatized, wondering if it meant a return to the old normal of worrying whether they might lose the grounded version of their mother, if only temporarily. Mark would know how to cope, but he would revert to carrying that nagging worry—*Will she have a seizure*?—if I were out on my own for long stretches. And I would want to assure them all—kids, partner, family of origin, acquaintances, coworkers, even strangers on the street—that, yes, once a seizure is over, I *am* okay. I'm the same stable, levelheaded person I've always been.

Providing that reassurance is an intimidating, exhausting task, at least as depleting as having seizures. With a little luck, I'll never have to do it again. Imagining that reality feels like sailing effortlessly through the sky buoyed by the invisible energy of a hot air balloon and liberated from the responsibility of assuring others. I am elated to be freed from that weight. My life load has been immeasurably lightened.

That I am still more concerned about others' imagined reactions and judgments than the seizures themselves is a cockamamie equation that speaks to the challenges of living with a chronic illness. While grateful that I have seizures under control, I still long for others' increased compassion, courage, and acceptance in the face of people's varying physical abilities. I yearn for a culture that doesn't disparage, shame, or exclude people with chronic conditions to the point where they feel like living with their health issues is harder than life-threatening medical procedures.

Under the Microscope Again

I'd been a grant-writing consultant on and off for twelve years when I saw a near perfect job advertised in January 2019 in the MIT Office of Engineering and Outreach, OEOP. The position looked ideal as it was part-time, on staff at a program housed on campus.

Universities are reputed for stability and benefits in the nonprofit sector, so I'd watched for open jobs at local colleges for years. OEOP—which has since changed its name to MIT Introduction to Technology, Engineering, and Science, or MITES—offers out-of-school-time science, technology, engineering, and mathematics or STEM enrichment activities to under-resourced middle school and high school students. Since 2015, I'd had three gigs focused on programs with similar or related goals. I'd also served as parent representative on my kids' school's improvement council and parented a tween. Between my personal and professional experience, I was a strong candidate, so I applied.

Like many universities, MIT has an e-portal for resumés and cover letters with a long standardized online application. I hesitated when I got to the question asking whether I had a disability. The form laid out the definition of disabled, and I clearly met it. I hadn't had a seizure for more than three years, but I had a history of them.

Should I admit to it? Haunted by my MEDUSA experience, I was tempted to answer no. I'd gone seizure-free long enough, and I could get away with concealing that information. But perhaps being honest would work to my advantage—maybe MIT had quotas they wanted to meet for numbers of staff with disabilities.

The application question included a standard disclaimer stating they didn't discriminate based on disability status. *Could I trust that?*

I wasn't sure. I saved the question for last. When I circled back to it, I decided it was best to tell them who I really was. I checked the yes box, hit submit, and hoped my choice wouldn't backfire in some way.

Within three days, an MIT HR recruiter reached out to arrange a phone interview. I'd applied for jobs there previously, so I knew it was only the initial step, the recruiter was the gatekeeper. With my strong fundraising background in out-of-school time programs, I handily got through the gate to MITES's finance and administration manager, and we arranged an interview for a week later. I began to stress out.

I tamped down my anxiety with extensive interview preparation. The finance administration manager informed me I would be interviewed by four identified people. Before the meeting day, I created a Word document with a mini biography about each of the interviewers. In addition to professional background, I knew where they went to college and grad school, when they graduated, and whether they volunteered anywhere.

I was an online troll. *Would any of them conduct the same level of research about me*? If so, they'd see the article I'd had published online the previous summer about the Americans with Disability Act, which mentioned my surgery and epilepsy. *Would they read that and make presumptions about me? Would anybody mention it during the interview?* I thought the answer to the last question was no, but I practiced a response.

The other thing I fretted about was my hair and whether to wear it up or down. I could dampen and twist it into a chignon with a colorful duckbill clip, so the curls sat atop my head, or I could pull most of it back into a ponytail and contain it with a short scarf tied into a decorative bow. Both styles somewhat tame my tresses, so I think of them as more conservative and businesslike. I often wear my hair pulled back or up during summer to keep cool, but in the middle of winter, when the interview would take place, I rely on it to help keep warm. More importantly, wearing my hair down looks better and allows me to present a more genuine version of myself.

When I trolled during interview prep, I noted from photos of them that three out of the four people who would interview me were African American women with curly hair. I decided odds were decent that fellow curly heads wouldn't hold my looser hair arrangement against me. I wore my hair down.

My in-person interview took place on a blah gray day, the cold air biting. I'd styled my hair carefully. Curls evenly framed my face on either side and, thanks to hair products and careful coiffing, the tresses on top defied gravity and held their shapes. I wrapped a giant scarf around my face and ears for warmth and, hat free, took the subway to Kendall Square.

I arrived excessively early to give myself time to scope out the campus and find my destination. Then I holed up in a nearby coffee shop until about fifteen minutes before the appointed time. I wanted to be timely but not crazy early. I arrived and introduced myself to the receptionist.

"I'll tell Faith you're here," she replied. Bright from natural light, the room had cubicles in the middle and small offices tucked in the corners. I took stock of the contents of my bag as I waited. I had a notebook, references, the list of foundations I'd come up with as best matches for MITES's mission, and writing samples. At one, the MITES manager of finance and administration fetched me.

"How are you doing today?" Faith asked as she led me to the conference room.

I lied and told her I was fine, but I was nervous as hell. Her colloquial manner put me somewhat at ease. I followed her to a windowless room with a large table in the middle and bright pink walls, one of which held a large white board.

"You're going to meet with Eboney first, our executive director," said Faith. "Then with John, the leadership giving officer from the school of engineering. After that, I'll return with Reimi—she's the program manager—for the final interview. I'll get Eboney now."

A moment later Faith walked in with Eboney. Eboney was medium height with tawny brown skin the color of café au lait, and true to the photo, she had long tightly curled tresses worn down that day. Based on my trolling, I knew she was around forty.

"I'm Eboney," she said as she shook my hand and I stood to greet her. Her wide smile lit her broad features. We sat down at the conference table, Eboney at the head, me one seat over.

"Let's start by having you walk me through your resume," she said, "so I can get a sense of your professional background." From that point, the meeting easily flowed as did the subsequent interviews. They asked standard questions about specific experience and skills—some of them multiple times. Given all the recent fundraising I'd done for out-of-school-time programs, I could eloquently speak to their importance. I shared my list of potential funders with Eboney, and she recognized some. I handed off my writing samples to the leadership giving officer.

Later, when Faith and Reimi asked what drew me to the position, I explained my role at the kids' school as both representative on the improvement council and as a parent of a middle-schooler and could genuinely relate my experiences back to the importance of out-of-school-time programs.

"The student body at my daughter's school has the biggest wealth gap of all six schools in Somerville," I explained. "The students aren't sophisticated enough to put words to it, but they're aware of it. They know there are haves and have nots, and it negatively impacts social dynamics. I had to transfer my son to a different school in Somerville because of social challenges he faced, and I know it was related to that dynamic. Programming like MITES's is great, because it gives under-resourced kids opportunities they wouldn't otherwise have."

I interviewed for more than three hours, which I took to be a good sign. Also, I noted that there had been good rapport-even some laughing—at different points in the afternoon. If anybody had read my published article about ADA, they didn't mention it.

At the end, Eboney came back in to say goodbye and go over last details. "How are you doing?" she asked me. I'd just returned from a quick bathroom break, where I was relieved to see my curls holding up.

"I'm pretty good—made it through the afternoon without getting flathead," I joked, which drew a smile from Eboney.

She collected my references and went over some last details before I left. Faith reached out to me within a week. I was excited when I saw the number flash on the cellphone—*It could be a job offer.* But, no, she was calling to inform me that they changed the job title from grant analyst to grant writer, and I had to reapply.

Pinging cartoony disappointment noises rang through my head—think SpongeBob SquarePants—as Faith explained. It wasn't all bad news, though. When they changed the job title, they raised the salary a little.

She instructed me to reapply through the MIT website but assured me I wouldn't have to go through a second interview. *Phew*!

I reapplied for the job the next day. I could write Faith's name where they asked if somebody at MIT told me to apply.—*That should help, right*? Again, I deliberated when I got to the question about whether I had a disability. *Yes or no*?

I looked up the language of the Americans with Disabilities Act, ADA. Signed into law in 1990, the ADA defines disability as "a physical or mental impairment that substantially limits one or more major life activities" and disabled as describing "a person who has a history or record of such an impairment, or a person who is perceived by others as having such an impairment." My epilepsy met the definition, even with the seizures under control.

When I'd come across the question on previous job applications, I'd reflexively answered no. I never thought my complex partial seizures limited my life activities. But after MEDUSA required me to fight them to prove my worth, I realized that, yes, my medical condition had impaired my ability to hold that job.

With the disruptive piece of my brain removed, I no longer worried about possible seizures taking over my body and subsequently forcing me to explain to others. I could choose whether to tell people I have epilepsy. My new invisible status granted me the privilege of opting to check no on the MIT application. I felt grateful for the camouflage provided by the ultimate success of my brain surgeries, but many other people were not so lucky.

I reflected on interactions with former colleagues, staff members at the kids' school, and even my own family members. Although the ADA provided a critical tool to my fight against workplace discrimination, it had done little to change others' perceptions of my disability, a shift achieved with brain surgeries. The ADA goal of assimilation into mainstream life cannot be achieved without a major cultural shift—one that equips people to accept that physical abilities of human beings vary. Based on my experience, nothing could provide a blueprint for it, as it requires something much larger than the provisions of the ADA—an increase in people's tolerance, empathy, and courage.

I turned my attention back to the MIT application and checked the yes box. As I formally owned up to vulnerability, I felt stronger. If quotas implied advantage, I'd damned well earned it. Presenting myself genuinely seemed to have worked so far, and the hiring team might not even see the form. Years later, I learned that hiring managers don't review initial application forms, but at the time, I thought that even if they did, the interviews had gone well enough that my answer wouldn't affect the outcome.

Within two weeks, Faith called to offer me the job.

❧❧

When I accepted the MITES position, my work commitment increased from twenty-five hours a month to twenty hours per week, almost triple the time, and I returned to an on-site office. While I lamented the loss of free time, I liked working outside the house. The position was a good fit both personally and professionally.

I reported directly to both Faith and Eboney, who had yin and yang management styles. Faith was quiet but strong and eager to offer guidance. As finance administrator, she was responsible for budgets, which meant that when we submitted grant proposals, she reliably provided all the financial information. I loved the arrangement, as I could spend most of my time writing grants and not hunting down figures. Eboney was an effervescent firebrand. She spoke passionately about MITES programs and inspired her audience whether comprised of students or donors. They were both competent leaders from whom I could learn something.

❧❧

About a year after I started, I was due for my annual review. By then, I'd established solid footing with my managers, colleagues, and the work. My significant experience and enthusiasm for the MITE's mission, combined with MIT's established brand, gave me a strong handle on grant writing. Nevertheless, as my review date approached, I felt anxious because MIT's employee evaluation process reminded me of MEDUSA's. They both started with a written self-assessment of my job responsibilities that I submitted to management. Then management wrote their own evaluations of my work, and everybody met to discuss the documents. When I went through the process at MEDUSA, it resulted in my threatening an ADA suit and ultimately losing my job. I thought I'd had a good first year at MITES, and most of my MITES colleagues didn't know I had epilepsy. I felt certain that the evaluation would have quite a different outcome.

I pushed back my fears and prepared my self-eval by reviewing my work for the year. It was a comforting exercise. I counted reports and proposals submitted and added up dollars raised, all impressive. Based on sheer numbers, I'd done a good job, yet I still felt anxious.

A positive MITES assessment would validate my professional worth, confirmation I desperately needed after my unjust and unrelated experience at MEDUSA. I coached myself repeatedly by remembering that what happened at MEDUSA had no bearing on my situation at MITES. Although my fears were irrational, I wanted that evaluation meeting over and done with.

The review took place in the same conference room as my interview. I waited nervously for my managers to join. The wait brought me back to MEDUSA meetings where Katherine flung my supposed inadequacies at me and accused me of looking spacey during meetings. Did I have an unknown lurking shortcoming my managers would soon lob my way?

Faith and Eboney joined me at the conference table. Despite my apprehension, I felt calmer than I had been on my MITES interview day. By evaluation day, I knew the people in the room, and we'd been working well together for a year. I was under a magnifying glass for both the review and the interview, but I had a year's worth of results for them to examine.

Eboney launched the meeting.

"I want to start by thanking you for all your hard work and the effort you brought to the team this year. When I read through your self-assessment, it was really helpful to see everything outlined like that."

Score. Thanks to the spreadsheet skills I'd cultivated, in part by keeping scrupulous medical records, drafting that section had been easy. *Okay, off to a good start. Now, would there be any curveballs? Any surprise complaints from a colleague? Some bigger unanticipated deficiency?*

"We hired you last year because we thought you'd elevate our grant submission efforts," Faith said. "I believe you succeeded at this, and I can honestly say it's a pleasure to supervise you."

I released some of the tension I had been holding in my shoulders. I murmured something appreciative, my quiet tone hiding my excitement and relief. There would be no false accusations tossed at me that day, only confirmation of what I knew was true: I was a valuable player on my team.

The rest of the meeting flowed smoothly enough. We discussed progress I'd made on specific goals I'd created, agreed upon strategic changes I could make, and established some simple new protocols to ensure clearer communication and workflow. Faith and Eboney identified a couple areas I needed to improve but nothing I couldn't easily address, nothing that felt unjustified, and certainly, nothing connected to my epilepsy. The review had a radically different upshot compared to what went on at MEDUSA. I got what I wanted—what any employee would want—an assessment based solely on my professional abilities and acknowledgement of my contributions.

I left the office looking forward to the short family vacation I would take in three days. With the review successfully behind me, I would enjoy it that much more. On the way home, I recalled Eboney using the phrase "your beautiful words" to describe a draft proposal I'd recently written, and it made me smile. The review confirmed what I suspected, that my managers valued and appreciated my work. The validation put a skip in my step as, picturing the beach in Puerto Rico, I walked home from Davis Square.

By chance, my longtime buddy and former MEDUSA colleague Robin would be in Puerto Rico at the same time. I looked forward to catching up with her family and enjoying some fun in the sun together. I also wanted to share news of my MIT evaluation with her.

"I had my first annual review at work last week, and it went really well." I was bursting with pride. "I was super nervous going into it—MIT's evaluation process is a lot like MEDUSA's, so it took me back. I was expecting the worst, but actually, it couldn't have gone better." We lay on the beach, a breeze drifting over us and the bright sun looming above warming the expansive sandy seaside.

"That's good," Robin said, looking out at the water where her son bobbed on a wave. Her response felt subdued compared to my sense of pride and relief. She didn't grasp the depth of my pre-evaluation apprehension. We'd been friends over thirty years, and she was my only MEDUSA colleague who knew all the details about what I'd been through.

I looked at Robin distracted by her son and watching gentle waves roll in. Despite our history, closeness, and her confidence, I'd gone through MEDUSA's bigoted ringer alone. The experience had occurred more than a decade before, and by the time we sat on the beach in Puerto Rico, I felt its effects only internally. Despite anything Katherine or MEDUSA claimed, professionally I was exactly where I wanted to be.

Removing the Weight

About six months after my emergency craniotomy I felt overjoyed despite slogging through adjustments in medication. Feeling both healthy enough to get out as much as I wanted and confident that the merry-go-round ride of grand mal week was behind me, I was elated. I sensed there was a good chance I wasn't going to have another seizure. Delighted by that that new conviction, I began singing to myself spontaneously as I ran my errands.

I'd walk around the neighborhood singing my off-key versions of songs that my musician friend calls comfort food music. Music and lyrics from tunes I frequently heard during childhood were indelibly ingrained in my brain. My repertoire comprised songs from the albums my parents played when I was a little girl. As a young adult, I bought them as CDs and played them for myself. Three Dog Night's "Joy to The World," Bob Dylan's "Blowin' in The Wind," and Sam Cooke's "Twistin' the Night Away" number among my all-time favorites, but during that healing phase, The Band's "The Weight" resonated loudest.

Written by Robbie Robertson, the song describes his visit to Nazareth, Pennsylvania. The song dedicates a verse to each of the buddies he visits: Crazy Chester, Miss Moses, Luke, Anna Lee, and Carmen. But it's the repetitive chorus about Miss Fanny that I relate to most. The singer implores that "a load" be removed from Miss Fanny and transferred to him. I was Miss Fanny walking around carefree with my happy secret that, although I still have epilepsy, I no longer have seizures. In addition to the liberation that comes with seizure-freedom, I was released from the obligation of explaining my disorder to others and managing their reaction to it. An immense freeing that empowered me to sing out loud even when Amelia begged me not to, that unshackling made a huge difference in my outlook.

"Mom, stop! That's embarrassing," she'd say as I belted out a tune while walking up the block.

"What do you care? There aren't even any other people on the sidewalk!" And I'd go back to my singing.

I equally identify with the singer accepting Miss Fanny's load during the song. Now that my medical condition is invisible to others, I am super aware of how privileged I am to have what appears to be a normal body. But I know what it's like to manage others' fears, intolerance, and judgment in the face of my body's imperfections.

Call to Action

With more than 50 million people affected globally by epilepsy, it ranks as the most common serious chronic brain disorder in the world. The 2022 National Institute of Health, NIH, made allocations for research of $212 million for epilepsy, $249 million for Parkinson's disease, and $3.3 billion for Alzheimer's disease and related dementias.

Considering that 3.4 million Americans have epilepsy, about a million have Parkinson's, and 5.8 million have Alzheimer's/dementia, funding amounts are disproportionate. For every American with epilepsy, NIH invests $62 into research. That number is $249 for Americans with Parkinson's and $569 for those with Alzheimer's/dementia. When it comes to money, epilepsy is the neglected stepchild disease.

Of the 50 million people with epilepsy, the United States Centers for Disease Control estimate that 3.4 million live in America. Thirty percent of them have uncontrollable seizures. That's a lot of people facing difficult situations and making tough decisions impacted by epilepsy.

My firsthand experience of the challenge inspired me to launch my blog in spring 2022 at lauraberetsky.com. Every month, I write about an online epilepsy-related news story, so I frequently come across new relevant research studies. Since I began blogging, I read about a study that used electroencephalogram, EEG, technology to detect seizures thirty minutes before they occur. I learned about the development of noninvasive brain surgery techniques that allow surgeons to remove a patient's faulty brain circuits without slicing their heads open. Oregon State University is developing a sensor system that enables patients taking carbamazepine to test their drug levels at home using their own saliva. *Wow!* I thought. *These developments would be so helpful to people who have uncontrollable seizures. I wish they were around when I still had them!*

I want to do a Snoopy dance when I read about cutting-edge advances, but I know they're in their infancy stages. It will be years before approval of new technology and before hospitals across the country widely use them, and longer before hospitals around the world employ them. More funding for epilepsy research will get new helpful technologies into the hands of people with uncontrollable seizures more quickly. Additional funding can also result in increased awareness and education, critical to ending discrimination against those with epilepsy.

Reaction to epilepsy has an especially sordid history. During European medieval times, physicians saw epilepsy as the result of demonic possession and treated people with epilepsy as witches and warlocks. Many women with epilepsy in Europe and colonial America died at the stake. People commonly believed epilepsy contagious and transmitted through the patient's breath. Thanks to medical advances and research, such practices and beliefs have been largely dispelled in the U.S.

Still, myths about epilepsy persist elsewhere in the world. In some under-resourced countries, many people believe the causes of epilepsy are related to witchcraft, atonement for sins committed by forebearers, or possession by supernatural forces. Instead of seeking solutions based on science and medicine, people look for traditional healers who use herbal remedies, rituals, spiritual curses, or combinations of them to address epilepsy Some methods can result in long-term health complications. For example, scarification with unsterilized sharp piercing instruments can lead to infections such as tetanus.

While we rely on medicine and science to treat epilepsy more consistently in the United States, stigmas persist. Some consider people with epilepsy strange, weird, or dangerous—generally someone to avoid.

Please take a moment and go to lauraberetsky.com and click on Readers in Action to donate to epilepsy research. Thank you.

Acknowledgements

Some say writing a book is like having a baby—it's a labor of love. Perhaps, although the gestation period for my book lasted literally eight times longer than for each of my children. Writing a memoir reminded me of running the Boston marathon, which I've never done. I expect you need to pace yourself and keep your energy steady, to make it to the finish line. Seeing my a book to publication required a marathoner's perseverance.

Seeing a book to publication resembles child-raising in that it takes a village of supporters to get a story from ideas in one's head to words on the page to a book readers hold. I will want to acknowledge all who supported me on my publication journey.

Thanks to Marcia Gagliardi, publisher at Haley's, for faith in my book. I am grateful for support provided as the book neared publication.

Thanks to the Grub Street Writing Center in Boston, where I took many memoir-focused classes. Specific shoutouts to instructors Nadia Colburn, Ethan Gilsdorf, and Judah LeBlang who read early versions of memoir sections and provided useful feedback. I am also grateful for Grub Street editors Michelle Seaton who helped me craft a book structure, Lynne Griffin who provided feedback on an early draft of the entire manuscript, and Katrin Schumann who helped me draft a query letter.

Additional gratitude to Allison K. Williams of the Writers' Bridge for early editing assistance and platform-building advice. And thank you to Jackie Vlahos for helping me implement my platform with website design assistance and savvy.

A second shoutout to Judah LeBlang for offering the Memoir in Progress class in fall 2017 that brought together some twelve students for ten weeks. When the course ended, six of us launched the Page Six Writers Group that has met regularly since. We provide feedback on sections of our emerging books and share writing journeys with each other. Page Six is alive and well today. A special thank you to each Page Sixer who cheered me on and kept me accountable to my story: Jean Duffy, Marcie Kaplan, Maggie Lowe, Susan Schirl Smith, and Bev Boisseau Stohl. I couldn't have completed the race without their support and encouragement.

Sincerest appreciation to Dr. Steven Schachter for writing the book's foreword and for serving as a leader in amplifying epilepsy patients' voices.

Gratitude to my son Liam for taking the pictures I used for my website and book promotion and to my daughter Amelia for providing the Medusa rendition for chapter headings.

Thanks to my sister Greta Beretsky-Disch for her suggestion of using our mother's artwork on the book cover. Special acknowledgement to my mother, Susan Gershon, who agreed to let me use it. Her wholehearted response moved me: "Of course you can. You are inspirational."

Thanks to my friends who served as beta readers for particular chapters: Faye Dupras, Pamela Goldstein, the late Christina Replogle, and Laurie Rosenblum. These pages reflect their invaluable feedback.

Writing about my seizures was sometimes tricky as I had frequently blanked out when I had them. Many seizure scenes include details supplied by family and friends with me at the time—in some cases decades ago. Thanks for such assistance to Greta Beretsky-Disch, Stanley Beretsky, Susan Gershon, Pamela Goldstein, Mark Jewell, the late Marcy Kagan, Michelle Plourde-Littlefield, Moragh Ramage, and Peter Walsh.

I am grateful to the neurology providers who supported my quest for excellent brain health. They include physicians from Boston's Brigham and Women's neurosurgery department and Brigham and Women's neurology team as well as researchers at California's Andrews Reiter Center. Although the meditation and breathing techniques I learned at the Andrews Reiter Center didn't control my seizures, to this day I use them to navigate through post-surgery neuroblips.

Guiding and advising me about the best steps to manage my epilepsy, Brigham and Women's neurology staff has provided my neurological care since 1988. While I sometimes questioned my neurologists' recommendations, I always felt confident in their expertise. Dr. E is my fifth neurologist at Brigham. While I imagine she found me irritable during my difficult recovery period, we both stuck it out. Now, with an annual check-in often via Telehealth, I'm likely one of her low-maintenance patients, a status I relish.

Thanks to my family of origin who raised me to be courageous, resilient, and logical. Had I not been brought up with those traits, the seizures may have gotten the better of me or held me back from achieving life goals. I grew up in an era that had less awareness of epilepsy and fewer resources for people with epilepsy and their families. My family did a great job caring for me while plowing through their own fears about a mysterious, sometimes scary condition. Thanks also for supporting me and my family during my post-surgery bummer of a summer.

Finally, enormous gratitude to my husband and children for supporting me while I worked on *Seizing Control*, putting up with additional babysitting, and postponement of other plans so I could write. Most importantly, great appreciation for bravely standing by me through seizures and surgeries. Although he didn't anticipate brain surgeries in the cards, my husband, Mark Jewell, had some idea of what he was getting into when he chose to marry and create a family with a person with epilepsy. Mark's optimism got me through double surgeries and my most challenging health recovery. Words cannot express my appreciation. I love you.

My son and daughter, Liam and Amelia Beretsky-Jewell, had no choice but to be raised by a mom with epilepsy. As Amelia astutely pointed out when she was eleven, it was a selfish choice on my part. My decision left my kids no choice but to face my seizures during their early childhood—they stepped up to the plate with impressive and touching bravery. I'm eternally grateful to them and forever sorry for any traumatizing impacts witnessing my seizures had on them as young children. While I know those are real, my confidence in our family's ability to overcome them outweighed my concerns. I am so proud of their courage, and I cherish watching them both mature into young adults.

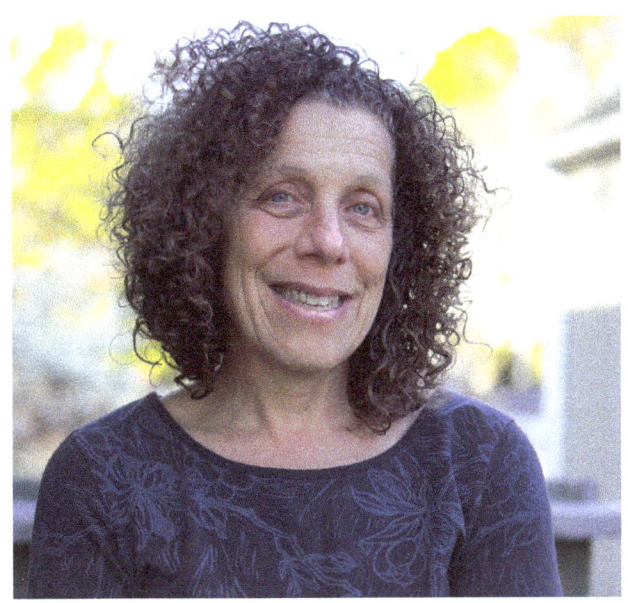

Laura Beretsky

About the Author

Laura Beretsky is a writer and community activist. She lives in Somerville, Massachusetts with her husband, children, and two cats where she's active on the local community preservation committee and high school parent-teacher-student association. She is a part-time grant writer at the Massachusetts Institute of Technology Introduction to Technology, Engineering, and Science department. Her writing has appeared in publications of the Health Story Collaborative and the National Library of Poetry and broadcast on the *Cognoscenti* section of radio station WBUR Boston. Her website at is lauraberetsky.com/

Resources

The most important resource for a person with epilepsy is an excellent neurologist. Epilepsy patients with complicated cases should find a neurologist who specializes in epilepsy, aka an epileptologist. Who needs an epileptologist? Patients with seizures medication can't control, those who have negative medication side effects, patients with other conditions that impact their epilepsy, and those pregnant or planning to become pregnant. Data shows that one in five people with epilepsy has active depression and twenty-six percent have anxiety disorders compared with eight percent and nineteen percent, respectively, of the general population. Couple such statistics with the thirty percent of us who have or had seizures that medication and other criteria listed can't control, and that's a lot of people who should work with an epileptologist.

Unfortunately, finding an epileptologist can be difficult. A quick search on MD.com found epileptologists in only thirty-three of fifty states. While WebMD.com lists them in all fifty states, many rural regions have epileptologists only in one major city. Since many people with epilepsy can't drive, that means a critical type of care may be inaccessible to those who live far from metro areas. Despite the complexity of epilepsy, telehealth appointments occur more often since the pandemic. I encourage those in need of an epileptologist's expertise to seek it out and meet virtually if necessary. A good epileptologist will know about latest research and innovations. Such skills and care can be life changing and lifesaving.

In addition to quality medical care, those with epilepsy need emotional support. The following list of resources includes online platforms where people with epilepsy communicate with one another.

Managing epilepsy can leave us feeling isolated, and connecting with others familiar with the challenges can provide valuable validation. This list is not comprehensive nor do listed resources substitute for good medical care.

Brain Ablaze Support Groups at brainablaze.com/epilepsy-support-group/pst-epilepsy-support-group-session/

Facilitated by David Clifford, an individual with epilepsy, Brain Ablaze meets held once a month via Zoom. People from around the world attend, mostly from the US and England. In an informal format, attendees introduce themselves, and the facilitator offers the opportunity to discuss epilepsy-related issues. Zoom meeting links are on the website.

Epilepsy Foundation of America
About Us | Epilepsy Foundation

The largest American epilepsy-focused nonprofit, EFA's mission involves fighting to overcome the challenges of living with epilepsy, accelerating therapies to stop seizures, and saving lives. With local chapters in forty-three states, EFA offers support groups, educational materials, trainings and funding for epilepsy research.

Phyllis Feiner Johnson's Epilepsy Talk Newsletter
epilepsytalk.com/

Phyllis Feiner-Johnson, who has had epilepsy for decades, advocates for those with epilepsy. She posts a monthly newsletter on medical issues that impact people with epilepsy.

My Epilepsy Team
myepilepsyteam.com/

My Epilepsy Team offers an online platform where people from all over the world with epilepsy maintain profiles, choose teammates, and post questions to and from each other.

Living Well with Epilepsy
livingwellwithepilepsy.com

Founded and managed by Jessica Keenan Smith, who has epilepsy. The site provides informational blogs, updates on epilepsy,-related news, and a regular newsletter with tips on navigating epilepsy-related challenges.

Andrews-Reiter Research Center
andrewsreiter.com/index.html

Dedicated to research and treatment of epilepsy, Andrews-Reiter Center's mission involvesresearching behavioral methods for improving seizure control. The center provides behavioral treatment techniques to individuals with intractable seizures. According to the website, some fifty percent of their patients attained full seizure control using these methods.

Facebook Discussion Pages

A moderator lightly monitors Facebook discussion pages and requires participants to complete a form prior to joining. Participants use the platform to share stories and seek advice about challenges of epilepsy. Facebook groups should never replace quality medical care.

Adults with Epilepsy/Seizures 40+: facebook.com/groups/1625582981015748

Defeating Epilepsy: facebook.com/groups/165011810757979

Epilepsy Awareness: facebook.com/groups/432316820139330

Epilepsy Awareness and Seizure Support Group: facebook.com/groups/2188155021436521

Epilepsy Global-Chat, support, advice: facebook.com/groups/epilepsysupports

Epilepsy/Seizure Support and Discussionfacebook.com/groups/101757649912249

Epilepsy Seizures/Let's Discuss It facebook.com/groups/EpilepsyAwarenessGrp

continued next page

Epilepsy Support Group:
facebook.com/groups/619401834741197
Now What Epilepsy Support Group, managed by the Cameron
Boyce Foundation:
facebook.com/groups/thecameronboycefoundation
Seizures Understanding and Support:
facebook.com/groups/SeizuresUnderstandingandsupport

Colophon

Text for *Seizing Control* is set in Bookmania, a font designed in 2011 by Mark Simonson to combine the sturdy elegance of the original Bookman Oldstyle, 1901, with the swashy exuberance of the Bookmans of the 1960s. With over 680 swash characters, more than any previous Bookman, the possibilities are endless. The broad range of weights make it great for display use, but it also works well for text. Unlike some Bookman revivals, it retains the original classic sloped roman for the italic. Bookmania includes all the features you would expect in a modern digital font family.

Title are set in Gill Sans, a humanist sans-serif typeface designed by Eric Gill and released by the British branch of Monotype from 1928 onwards. Gill Sans is based on Edward Johnston's 1916 Underground Alphabet, the corporate font of London Underground.

Milton Keynes UK
Ingram Content Group UK Ltd.
UKHW020609201123
432904UK00009B/164